MARIE OSMOND'S GREAT PROGRAM
TO GET YOU BACK INTO SHAPE—AND GIVE
BABY THE BENEFITS OF EXERCISE TOO!

Now you can get your body back in shape and have your baby benefit too! Marie Osmond's gentle, effective exercise program, developed by Elizabeth Noble, famous physical therapist and pregnancy/childbirth expert, is safe for mothers and their babies to begin just a few weeks after birth. Specific exercises target the muscles stressed by childbearing, and help restore them to pre-pregnancy perfection. Each routine, illustrated and including important warm-up exercises, provides stretching and strengthening that feel wonderful and flatten the tummy, tone up legs, hips, and buttocks, and relieve backaches from lifting and carrying Baby all day.

Best of all, carefully tested, playful infant exercises make Baby your partner in fun, and stimulate Baby's natural development. And a step-by-step guide to baby massage helps relax even a colicky infant. Babies love this program, with its body rhythms, happy movements, and close physical interaction with mother. The result is more than just a work-out—it's a wonderful way to further personal growth and build new bonds of love. You'll also find:
* Water and ball activities for Baby
* Professional tips on lifting and carrying Baby
* Infant development guidelines
* A guide to other resources

ELIZABETH NOBLE, a registered physical therapist, is a renowned pregnancy and childbirth expert and Director of the Maternal and Child Health Center in Cambridge, Massachusetts. She is the bestselling author of *Essential Exercises for the Childbearing Year, Having Twins, Childbirth with Insight,* and *Marie Osmond's Exercises for Mothers-to-Be* (also available from NAL Books).

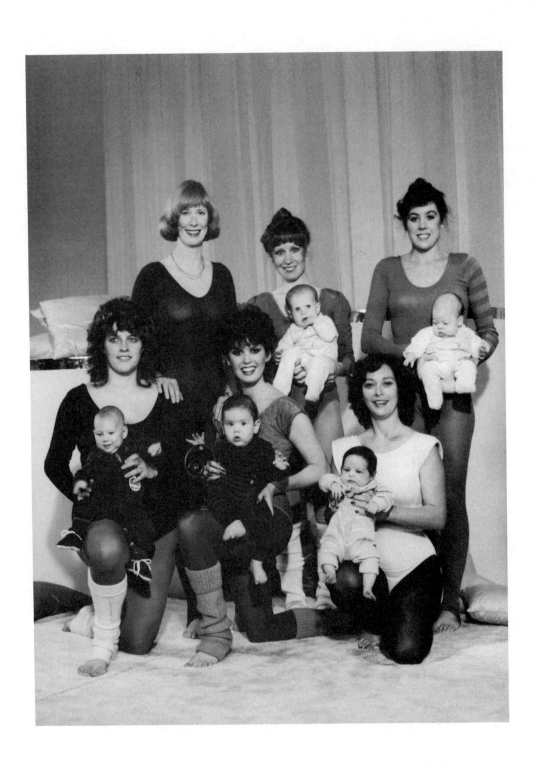

Marie Osmond's EXERCISES FOR MOTHERS AND BABIES

ELIZABETH NOBLE

NAL BOOKS

NEW AMERICAN LIBRARY

NEW YORK AND SCARBOROUGH, ONTARIO

Publisher's Note
The ideas, procedures, and suggestions contained in this book
are not intended as a substitute for consulting with your physician.
All matters regarding your health require medical supervision.

Published simultaneously in Canada by
The New American Library of Canada Limited.

 NAL BOOKS TRADEMARK REG. U.S. PAT. OFF. AND FOREIGN COUNTRIES
REGISTERED TRADEMARK—MARCA REGISTRADA
HECHO EN HARRISONBURG, VA. U.S.A.

SIGNET, SIGNET CLASSIC, MENTOR, PLUME, MERIDIAN AND NAL BOOKS
are published *in the United States* by New American Library, 1633 Broadway,
New York, New York 10019, *in Canada* by The New American Library of Canada
Limited, 81 Mack Avenue, Scarborough, Ontario M1L 1M8

Library of Congress Cataloging in Publication Data
Noble, Elizabeth, 1945–
Marie Osmond's exercises for mothers and babies.

Bibliography
Includes index.
1. Postnatal care.   2. Exercise for women.
3. Exercise for children.   4. Infants—Care and
hygiene. I. Title.
RG801.N63   1985   613.71   85-7273
ISBN 0-453-00486-5

Designed by Marilyn Ackerman

First Printing, October, 1985

1 2 3 4 5 6 7 8 9

PRINTED IN THE UNITED STATES OF AMERICA

To Linda Gallagher

Acknowledgments

The exercise program presented in this book is based on the Mother and Baby postpartum exercise class developed at the Maternal and Child Health Center in Cambridge, Massachusetts, which I direct.

My partner at the Center, Linda Gallagher, and Judy Friedman, both pediatric physical therapists, made major contributions to this program and compiled the Infant Development Guide on pages 26–27. I am especially grateful to Linda for her additions to the manuscript.

I wish to thank 3/West Productions, Inc, of Southfield, Michigan, which had the idea of bringing together a popular star and an obstetric physical therapist for home health education. The project was developed by Irving D. Goldfein and Rosalind Lullove Cooperman, executive producers of 3/West Productions, Inc., for MGM/UA Home Entertainment Group, Inc., as a sequel to the prenatal exercise program with Marie Osmond that was recorded on videotape by MGM/UA Home Entertainment Group, Inc., and 3/West Productions, Inc., in 1983, and published in book form as *Marie Osmond's Exercises for Mothers-to-Be* by New American Library in 1985.

The photography was done by Robert Brantley Photography, Salt Lake City, Utah. Roz Cooperman, also director of photography, organized the wardrobe and models. The set was designed by Seven Neilson, of the Osmond Studio in Orem, Utah. Special thanks are due to the Osmond Media Corporation, Orem, Utah, for their assistance.

I am also appreciative of the efforts of Ronna Wallace and Donna Bascom of MGM/UA and literary agent Connie Clausen, of New York, in helping to bring this exciting project to fruition.

I would like to express special thanks to Marie Osmond and her son, Stephen James, for their enthusiastic participation in this project. Thanks also to the other parents and babies who posed for photos: Michelle Baum and son Christopher Jeff; Michelle and Michael F. Lundell (parents of five) and daughter, Charlotte Elizabeth; Penny Cain and daughter, Megan Sheri; and Janice S. Goldfein and daughter, Ariella Rahel.

Contents

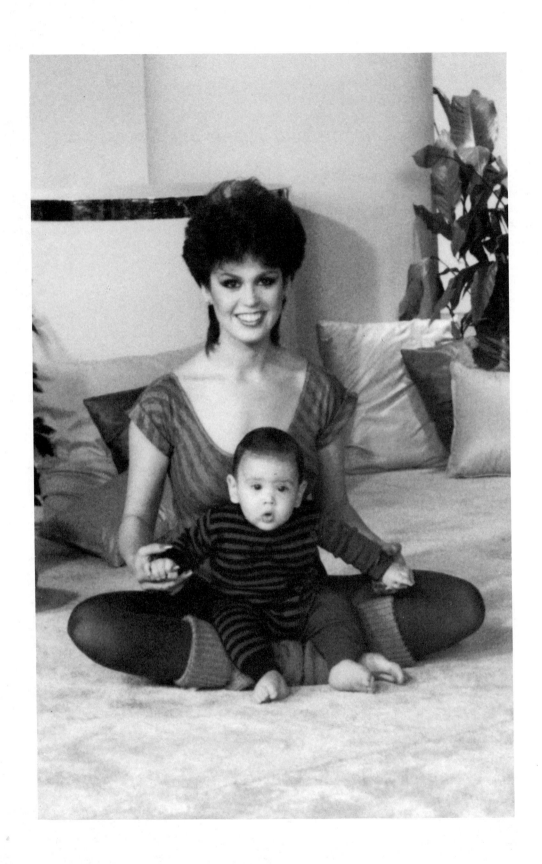

Marie's Foreword

Having and raising a baby is one of life's most wonderful experiences. Yet like me, I'm sure you want to get your body back in shape as soon as possible.

The great thing about this exercise program is that you can do just that and have your baby join in, too!

These exercises are so safe for you and your baby that you can start them in the first few weeks after the birth. They were designed by physical therapist Elizabeth Noble, who created my prenatal exercise program for a videotape and companion book, Marie Osmond's Exercises for Mothers-to-Be *(New American Library, 1985).*

Meeting Elizabeth Noble, an internationally known expert in exercise and health during and just after pregnancy, was one of the best things that could have happened to me and my baby Stephen.

The strength, flexibility, balance, coordination, and grace Elizabeth Noble's plan gave me during pregnancy carried over to my life after Stephen was born and made my postpartum recovery easier.

Elizabeth Noble's program for mother and child after birth is designed not only for maximum health and physical flexibility, but also to further the loving bond between a mother and her new infant. Gentleness—and affection—are at the heart of every exercise.

The program is based on the Mother and Baby exercise classes at the Maternal and Child Health Center which Elizabeth directs in Cambridge, Massachusetts. It makes me very happy to know that through this book you and your baby will be able to benefit from it just as much as Stephen and I have.

The concept behind Mother and Baby exercises is the enjoyable interaction between parent and child. So of course fathers are wel-

come to share in the fun too. In addition to the exercises there are also instructions for water and ball activities and infant massage.

This infant exercise system goes far beyond baby massage, however, because Elizabeth belongs to the increasing number of experts who believe in the importance of real exercise even for the youngest infant.

Let's face it, though. We need the exercise more than our babies! It's really important for us to strengthen the muscles affected by childbearing. We also need to work on our upper backs and arms, with all the lifting and carrying that we now have to do.

Yet often, we new mothers find we don't make that time for ourselves. Being a mother is a round-the-clock job!

That's why I know you'll love this program. It will become a special part of the day for you and your baby to enjoy each other as you both tone up your muscles. The movements and massage will also help your baby relax and sleep well.

So let's get going and have some fun with our babies!

—Marie Osmond

Introduction to Marie's Program

*T*he following postpartum exercise program is designed to meet the special needs of a new mother's body while enhancing the natural development of her infant.

Along with the other obstetric physical therapists at my private practice, the Maternal and Child Health Center in Cambridge, Massachusetts, I have taught this program to hundreds of mothers and babies over the past few years. The program is one of the most popular presentations that I give across the country to health-care professionals and to the media.

The exercises are safe, yet challenging, and very enjoyable for both mother and baby. You can start this program at any time, depending on how you feel after the birth. However, if you wait until two or three months have gone by, the baby is heavy for some of the lifting exercises. Ideally, you should start within a month after the birth and let your muscles develop as your baby's weight increases.

The muscles that you prepared for birth are the same ones that now require restoration. In this program, muscle groups are alternated so that no one group is overworked at any time. Stretches are done slowly because bouncing stimulates the muscle to tighten against the direction of movement. Prenatal exercises focusing on the abdominal and pelvic floor muscles are now incorporated into a larger context which also includes strengthening of the shoulders, arms, and upper back.

All the exercises in this book include the baby. In fact, part of what makes these movements and activities special is that they are safe for very young babies. Many mothers start our program when their babies are just a couple of weeks old.

At first, most new parents are unsure about their offspring's potential and need special inspiration and encouragement to interact more physically with their baby. Mothers and fathers become really excited when they see the enormous range of activities that they can enjoy with their child. So it is my great pleasure to have this opportunity to share with childbearing couples the mother and baby postpartum exercise program developed at the Maternal and Child Health Center.

As a physical therapist specializing in obstetrics and gynecology, I taught my first exercise class to pregnant women in 1965 in Australia, where I did my training. In the decade that I have lived in the United States, I founded the Obstetrics and Gynecology Section of the American Physical Therapy Association and have been active in promoting the role of exercise and physical therapy through the childbearing years. Over the years, I recognized a tremendous need for postpartum exercise programs that would also help the new mother to understand normal infant development and to enjoy her baby.

This program is presented to encourage you to get in touch with your own needs and those of your baby. For you—like every mother-infant pair—are unique.

Exercise after childbearing is about more than just physical improvement. It is an avenue of personal growth. Simply being aware of and facilitating your baby's growing skills will help to strengthen the bond between you and add to your self-esteem as a caring and competent parent.

—Elizabeth Noble

1

Your Body After Childbirth

Be patient with your body after childbirth.

During pregnancy, your abdominal muscles were stretched taut over your expanding uterus, but now that you have given birth, all that extra slack in the muscles has to be taken up. You will need to spend time shortening the stretched muscles before you can progress to strengthening them. Also, although your pelvic floor is not as low now as it was at the end of pregnancy, the muscles were stretched over the baby's head if you had a cesarean delivery, and it may take weeks or months before you regain full pelvic floor control.

The growth in breast size which you noticed in pregnancy increases even more when the milk comes in, about the third day after birth. Although breast size settles down when nursing is well established, the circumference of the chest remains enlarged for a few months, preventing you from buttoning those pre-pregnancy shirts.

The weight gained around the hips and thighs is a store of calories laid down for breastfeeding, and it usually takes several months to go away, especially since nursing mothers should not diet. On the contrary, you need five hundred more calories a day than you did during pregnancy because lactation is an even greater nutritional challenge to your body.

Some women spring right back into their former shape and weight very soon after the birth, but they tend to be the exception. For most of us, it takes at least three to six months, and sometimes more, so be patient. While actual weight loss may take months, however, there is no reason why you cannot restore your muscles to normal tone and strength within weeks.

Restoring Muscle Tone and Strength

The Abdominal Muscles   The abdominal muscles are the most obvious group in need of restoration after birth. Most women gaze in dismay at their

15

flabby belly and loose skin. Because the abdominal muscles support your spine, they must be in good shape to protect your back for the months and years of lifting Baby that lie ahead.

The abdominals are structured like a layered corset, enabling you to move your trunk and pelvis in different directions. The outermost muscles of the abdomen run vertically on each side of your navel and are called the recti muscles. These two muscles join in a fibrous band running down the midline of your abdominal wall. (You may have noticed this central indentation in athletes or weight lifters.)

The hormonal softening of the body tissues that occurs in pregnancy, along with the stretching of the abdominal muscles and the stress of childbirth, can cause this "center seam" to separate. Everyone has a gap of about an inch. However, if you can fit three or more fingers into the gap, you will need to do a corrective exercise to bring the muscles parallel before beginning abdominal exercises that involve curling up your head and shoulders, lowering both your legs. These steps are outlined in Chapter 6, Exercises on Your Back.

Cesarean mothers have an even greater need to regain muscle tone and strength in the abdominal wall. The surgery, pain, and incision cause a greater delay in the return of muscle strength than after a vaginal birth, so exercises are essential. Abdominal exercises will also help to prevent the gas pain that occurs after abdominal surgery.

The Pelvic Floor   The pelvic floor is a band of muscles which is attached like a hammock across the bottom of your pelvic cavity. These muscles are usually the muscles most affected by childbearing. Even if you had a cesarean delivery, this muscular shelf still had to support the increasing weight of your baby during pregnancy. Hormones also made your pelvic floor soften and become more lax to help it stretch over the baby's head during birth. You need to exercise these muscles so they recover their strength and elasticity.

If you had a tear or an episiotomy (incision to enlarge the vagina during birth), pelvic floor exercises are even more important, for they must promote healing and good circulation in the sutured tissues.

Your pelvic floor muscles function in urine control, sexual response, and support of your pelvic organs. Control over these muscles is essential for female health and you should continue to exercise them for the rest of your life. It has been estimated that about half of all Caucasian women suffer from pelvic floor problems; much gynecological surgery is done to correct them. If you cannot stop your urine flow, or have ever had trouble retaining a diaphragm or tampon, you certainly need to improve your pelvic floor muscles.

For more details on pelvic floor and abdominal muscle function and treatment, and a special chapter on cesarean birth and recovery, refer to my book *Essential Exercises for the Childbearing Year* (see Recommended Reading).

Muscles for Lifting Baby   It is also important to build up your *arms, shoulders and back* for lifting and carrying Baby. Most women are weak in these areas and find it difficult, for example, to do even modified push-ups.

Many of the exercises in this program involve strengthening the back, shoulder girdle, arms, and wrists. The sooner you start these with your baby, the better, because if Baby grows too heavy before you start, then some of them may be too difficult. Fathers, on the other hand, always seem to be able to do the various baby lifts.

Lifting and carrying the baby is a central part of parenting, and plays an important role in Baby's experience of movement and body position.

Learning to Relax

Rest and relaxation are even more important for you now that you have to tend to the demands of your newborn in addition to recovering from the birth and adjusting to the many physical and emotional changes in your life.

Lying on your front with a pillow under your hips (put two under your hips and one under your chest if your breasts are tender) is a wonderful way to rest. It relieves pressure on vaginal stitches if you have any, and helps the spine regain its normal alignment. It is important for cesarean mothers to lie on their front as soon as possible, because the several days they spend in the hospital of half-lying with a rounded spine may lead to severe backache.

Getting the most out of this program is just a matter of working *with* your body rather than pushing it to extremes. You should feel rejuvenated after exercise, not exhausted. Feel free to go slowly and pause frequently to rest.

One of the benefits of this program is that you will be attending to your baby during all the exercises and enjoying his or her response. Rest pauses will help you to take a less compulsive and more relaxed view of exercise than you might have otherwise. Resting often will also help to prevent overstimulating your baby and avoid stiffness of your muscles.

Babies can learn to share quiet times as well as exercise activities. Often at the end of our class sessions at the Maternal and Child Health Center, there will be absolute silence in the room as all the mothers and babies relax to a tape of soothing music.

Remember, be patient in the beginning.

2

Your Baby's Physical and Emotional Development

Movement and its accompanying sensations are the foundation of all learning, identity, and emotional development. Babies develop social skills and self-esteem from refining their strength, mobility, and flexibility with their parents' encouragement.

The first weeks and months present an early opportunity to encourage your baby's natural abilities. Rocking, bouncing, swinging, and other rhythmical changes of Baby's position stimulate receptors in Baby's ears which help develop Baby's sense of position and motion. The combined movements you do in this exercise program help Baby begin to understand the meaning of right and left, up and down, backward and forward, here and there, close and far, high and low, stop and start.

It is important to point out, however, that normal babies do not need "exercises" for proper development, because they are programmed to develop naturally in a certain sequence. They learn to crawl, creep, sit, walk, and talk without any syllabus or examinations!

Make sure that you only *facilitate* the positions and actions of your baby, never forcing or pushing her to do the things she is not ready to do yet. This program offers ways to make the most of each stage of your baby's development, without trying to speed it up and mold a "superbaby." You don't want to assist your child so much that the challenge is removed.

A general timetable for infant development follows on pages 26–27. This is just to be used as a guide, however; do not expect your baby's milestones to conform precisely to this schedule. Like each birth, each baby is unique and will unfold with his or her own style and timing.

Holding Your Baby: The Veldman Technique

One of the most important aspects of your baby's physical and emotional development is the way you hold her.

Frans Veldman, the Dutch founder of Haptonomy (the science of touch and affectivity) has researched how mothers in different cultures around the world carry their infants. It is his strong recommendation that babies be held so that they are with a "haptonomic circle" with their caretaker, providing them with physical and emotional security. The following illustrations on page 20 demonstrate these supportive positions.

Note that in every case, the child is supported from the *base*. This is the heaviest part of the human body—the center of gravity. The pelvic area has great significance in certain Eastern cultures where it is considered to be a key location of a person's feelings. The Japanese call this area *hara,* and in yoga this second *chakra,* or energy center, is considered to be the seat of self-affirmation.

A child who through infancy is lifted, supported, and thus affirmed from this area, develops an expanded sense of his or her self through the body. According to Veldman, whose training includes medicine, physical therapy, and psychology, such a child is less likely to develop any of the common sexual, emotional, or orthopedic problems with the pelvis in adult life. In fact, Veldman's "hapto-psychotherapy" uses loving touch to treat psychologically disturbed adults in order to fulfill these needs not met in childhood. Veldman publishes in Dutch and French; however, interested readers can enquire about any future visits by Veldman to the United States by writing to the Maternal and Child Health Center in Cambridge, Massachusetts (see Resources).

A baby held from her base can and will hold her spine and head erect—from the moment of birth! Most people will not believe this because they are afraid to try it. By "protecting" the baby in a crumpled position, caretakers are actually fulfilling their own limited prophesy of the baby's postural abilities.

I should point out that mothers are usually terrified the first time I demonstrate this way of holding their baby. But as soon as parents try it and see their baby's contentment, they are immediate converts.

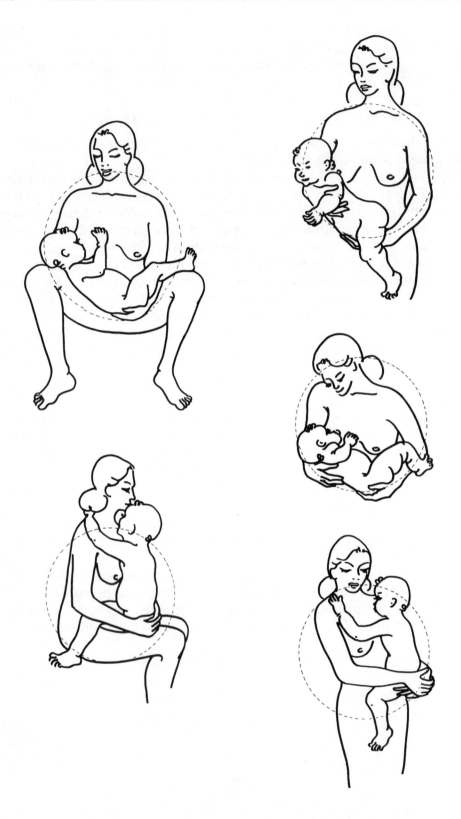

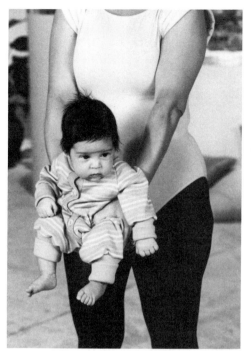
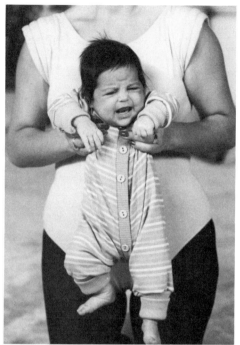

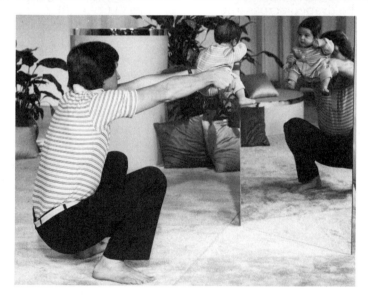

Held from her base, Baby observes her surroundings with poise and is able to move her trunk and arms freely. Lifted under her shoulders, Baby feels the alarming sensation of having her heaviest part dangling, putting even more strain on her armpits. Arm, head, and trunk movements are greatly restricted. Squashed in this way, the rib cage cannot expand, which interferes with Baby's breathing.

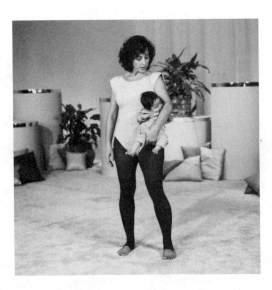

The emotional consequences of how Baby is held are just as important. Frans Veldman stresses the necessity to pick up, hold, and carry the baby in this way, affirming her independence and self-worth. Baby is not a sack of potatoes to be draped across one hip! Baby has every right to face and interact with the world, with just enough support (psychological and physical), but not too much.

At the Mother and Baby classes at the Maternal and Child Health Center, we see a difference in babies who are held in this way, especially when the parents have previously attended our childbirth classes and have understood the need to support the baby from its base beginning at the time of *birth*. These babies are calm and confident and show excellent head and trunk control in the first few weeks.

As Baby grows heavier, mothers often find that this increasing weight puts great strain on their wrists. Fathers, however, when encouraged to hold Baby in this way, enjoy it immensely and have the physical stamina to continue longer. An alternative is to pick Baby up between his or her legs, especially as a toddler or older child. Sometimes concern is expressed about lifting boys in this way, but there is no more pressure on the genitals for a male than riding a bike or lying on his front.

Body Contact

Babies need and enjoy a great deal of body contact with their parents— much more than most of them receive in our culture. Despite common misconceptions, increased body contact with your baby will enhance rather than discourage later independence.

Nursing, feeding, or exercising with your baby skin-to-skin, using a baby carrier instead of a carriage or stroller, and having the baby in the same bed with the parents, all offer extra body contact which strengthens your child's sense of security.

Skin-to-skin Benefits Allow your baby to be naked at times, especially in winter when she usually has to be heavily clothed. She will benefit from the tactile stimulation of being placed on different surfaces, such as your naked skin, a towel, velvet, carpeting, plastic, etc. An "air bath" also promotes healthy skin. Baby needs to feel his or her *whole* body; so even the diaper should be removed for at least some of the time. (You can keep it under Baby's bottom.)

Baby Carriers for Security Women from the beginning of time have always carried their babies on their bodies, providing warmth, security, and movement. In fact, in many cultures mothers can intuit when their babies need to pass wastes and diapers are not used. For such women, this is no different from feeling their own bodily needs, and they are disbelieving that modern mothers no longer have this skill.

In traditional cultures such as those in Africa, India, and South and Central America, women generally use just a length of cloth which they tie over one shoulder or above their breasts for a baby carrier. The cloth is versatile and can be folded around the baby's head and body as desired. The baby is always carried on the mother's back, which allows Baby to interact more with the world than she can from the front, where the view is only of Mother's chest.

Many mothers give up using modern baby carriers because of the aches and pains that arise in their backs and shoulders as Baby drags them forward. It is actually much more comfortable and efficient for your muscles if you carry the baby on your back, and this can be done from birth. For the first few weeks of life, infants' heads do wobble around—which may make adults unduly concerned. I always reassure parents of newborns that I have never seen a baby's head roll off!

In general, try to avoid all the baby furniture and appliances on the market today that serve to separate you physically from your infant.

Carrying the baby on your body is not only natural and simple, but it makes life so much easier for you, especially with a baby who is making it clear that it needs a lot more holding. If a baby is in frequent and prolonged physical contact with a parent, in those early months before the baby becomes mobile, all parties are secure with regard to each other's welfare.

Trying the Family Bed Humans (in modern times) are the only mammals who do not sleep with their young. Many parents are concerned about their baby while he sleeps and anxiously keep checking on him to make sure he is still breathing! How much simpler to have the babe snuggled up next to you. For parents who set their baby aside in a bassinet or crib, often in another room, the business of "putting the baby to sleep" may become a problem. This is never seen in families and cultures where the bed is shared. The infants and children are happy, confident, and self-regulating. Because the little ones have enjoyed warmth, security, and body contact through the night, during the day they are easy and independent.

By the same token, parents with a baby who demands to be held all the time might try the family bed to see if the extra body contact through the night satisfies their infant's need for touch and affirmation.

Those readers who have queries about parents and children sleeping together will find reassuring discussions of the practice in *The Family Bed*, by Tine Thevinen, and *The Continuum Concept*, by Jean Liedloff (see Recommended Reading.)

Stimulation

All of a newborn's senses are very acute. A baby's brain undergoes great development in its first year of life and he or she learns more at that time than in any successive year. Babies respond enthusiastically to singing, pantomiming, music, mobiles, parents' movements, their own image in a mirror, and other babies.

Baby is familiar with Mother's and Father's voices from before birth and enjoys conversation. From the beginning, always talk to your baby as if he or she understands, whether you are discussing what to buy in the grocery store, describing the clothes you are putting on his different body parts, or requesting him to cooperate with some activity you must do.

This approach is not only better for your baby's future speech development, but it is a sign of respect from you for your baby. As those readers who have studied a foreign language will know, understanding comes long before verbal mastery.

Self-Expression

Everyone would agree that all newborns have distinct personalities, yet many people find it hard to accept that the roots of personality are laid down in the uterine environment. Psychotherapies that bring about regression of an adult to his or her birth and prenatal memories have shown that this is indeed a crucially formative time.

Babies tend to behave outside the uterus in the way that they behaved inside with regard to their level and timing of activity. Sometimes the baby has a fussy period each day that corresponds to the time of birth, or perhaps the onset of labor. Babies who had a difficult birth, or who were not the gender their parents preferred, may need to do a lot of screaming to relieve their frustration.

Parents who see their child as a keenly aware, whole person can support their child's needs to express bad feelings as well as good ones. The baby massage you will learn in this book is a great help for "colicky" infants who become tense and scream for several hours a day, usually at the same time each day.

Self-Regulation

Babies come into the world with their own unique scripts. If parents can allow their baby to be a self-regulating being, they will reap this freedom back for themselves.

It is difficult to have the baby direct your life with regard to his sleeping and eating. Nursing mothers always comment that they never realized that the baby would eat so constantly, for the fantasy of a schedule still remains in the backs of our minds from harsher times of child-rearing.

Mothers who feel obliged to direct their baby's schedule and activities at all times usually suffer the same loss of self as the baby does in such circumstances. By "loss of self" I mean that Baby will be demanding and difficult, lacking in composure and the ability to be himself, by himself. As Boston pediatrician Berry Brazelton often points out, babies are able to manipulate all the adults around them!

Mothers who feel that their time and energy is totally sacrificed to the baby, come to feel that they can no longer be themselves either. This vicious cycle is much easier to prevent than to break, and readers will benefit from such books as *Birthrights*, by Richard Farson and *The Feeling Child*, by Arthur Janov (see Recommended Reading), which support parents' and children's need for intuition and spontaneity. We all learn to parent as we go along, and each of us must find our own harmonious path.

Enriched Potential

Many new parents are more anxious about and protective of their baby than necessary. One of the great benefits of this mother and baby exercise program is the increased confidence that occurs for both baby and parents as Baby gains strength and mobility, and Mother and Father see that Baby is not the fragile creature they feared.

Providing your baby with touch and movement experiences will enrich his or her potential for development. Baby is a sensual being from the moment of conception, and affirming Baby's sensuality enables healthy sexuality to develop. Encouraging your infant to enjoy a wide range of movement brings about increased confidence, coordination, and enjoyment of sport and exercise. These innate human skills need to be nurtured in our sedentary society where radio and television often provide all the singing, movement, and stimulation a child gets. Let today's parents resist this trend toward passivity and rear spontaneous and original children.

Approximate Infant Development Guide*

Birth to Six Months

Age	Movement	Vision	Sensation/Perception	Communication	Emotional/Social
Birth–1 mo.	Flexion position. Random movements. Grasps; hand to mouth.	Limited (7"–12").	Accommodates to stimuli and may fall asleep. Responds to touch.	Discomfort sounds. Grunts, gurgles.	Bonding with caretaker. Stops crying at human voice.
1–2 mo.	Turns head fully. Faces outstretched arm.	Stares; eyes point together.	Coordinates sound and sight.	Coos. Attends speaker.	Recognizes key persons. Quiets when picked up.
2–3 mo.	Lifts head when lying on front. Hand to mouth.	Looks at hands. Swipes at objects.	Moves toward touch. Follows sound with eye and head movement.	Can distinguish anger and approval sounds.	Smiles, attends to human face and voice.
4 mo.	Props on elbows. Rakes with hand. Feet to mouth. Rolls front to back.	Visually curious. Independent eye/head movement.	Senses sides. Reaches with one or both arms.	Responds vocally to sound.	Increased periods of responsiveness.
5 mo.	Props on extended elbows. Reaches. Holds object in both hands; some finger control.	Eye/hand and eye/foot coordination.	Grasps without looking. Aware when objects disappear from view.	Increased babbling sounds with both lips.	Anticipates daily events. Knows familiar things.
6 mo.	Lifts head when lying on back. Rolls from back to front. Begins to hold bottle.	Begins to distinguish figure from background.	Senses body in space.	Increased laughing and cooing.	Engages in solitary play.

* Courtesy of Linda Gallagher, R.P.T. and Judith Friedman, R.P.T.

Six to Twelve Months

Age	Movement	Vision	Sensation/ Perception	Communication	Emotional/Social
6–7 mo.	Learns to balance in sitting.	Eyes transfer from object to object.	Objects become permanent in memory.	Listens, quiets when name called. Understands simple function words.	May withdraw from strangers; moves to familiar person.
7–8 mo.	On front, pivots and pushes backward. Crawls on belly. Pats with open hand.	Looks for details.	Imitates. More aware that he causes effect.	Self-initiated babbling, repetitive. Vocal play imitation.	May develop fear of unknown.
8–9 mo.	Drive to erect posture, pulls to standing. Creeps on hands and knees. Bangs, throws, drops, squeezes.	Looks at spot being touched.	Anticipates body movement in song.	Starts to use symbolic gestures.	Waves. Shakes head.
9–10 mo.	Masters sitting. Cruises, side steps. Refined grasp. Turns wrist to open hand; finger-feeds.	Looks at self and recognizes others in mirror.	Coordinates both sides of body. Refined awareness of right and left. Examines 3-dimensional objects. Explores depth relationships.	Long and varied vocal sounds.	Refines style of response to situation. Assists with dressing; takes off.
10–11 mo.	Skilled creeping, changes direction. Walks with hand held. Falls to sitting. Manipulates 2 objects in 1 hand. Pokes, points.	Connects images with 3-dimensional objects. Interest in books. Searches for favorite toys.	Uses tools, pulls string. Simple construction (building blocks, etc). Aware of sensory characteristics (wet, chewy, etc).	Follows simple orders. Gives toys if asked. Realizes some sounds get more rewards. Says first function words and labels (9–18 months).	Increased curiosity. Realizes specific infant action gets adult reaction. Uses various actions to change results. Enjoys own competence.
11–12 mo.	Understands in/out, up/down, under/around/on. Refines grasp and finger function.	Scans picture books.	Begins trial and error. Uses objects functionally.	Use of jargon and intonation with babbling.	Motivated by internal gratification.

3

Tips for Exercising

The ideal time to start exercising *with Baby* is a couple of weeks after birth. You will be busy enough until then, recovering from the birth and establishing Baby's feeding.

If you had a cesarean delivery, you can begin *with Baby* at about one month postpartum, if you are in good general condition.

If your baby is, say, four or five months old already, begin to exercise with Baby right now. You both will gain a lot from the exercises as well as the interaction with each other. If you have never exercised before, just do each exercise a couple of times in the beginning since Baby will be a bit heavy for you to lift.

Work on your physical recovery whenever your baby's schedule permits. Simply exercise through the day as the opportunities arise. Most of the exercises described do not require any special equipment. Your living room rug is fine, or a blanket on the grass. You can do these exercises at the beach or even on your bed (although a harder, firmer surface is easier to work on).

Loose clothing for both of you is fine, and if conditions are warm enough, try doing the exercises skin-to-skin.

Here are some additional tips that will add to the pleasures and benefits of exercising with your Baby.

1. *Encourage Baby's participation, but do not force it.*

   In our classes at the Center, which last one and a half hours, no baby ever does all of the exercises in one session, because of naps, eating, diaper changes, or fussing. Fussy periods are amazingly rare in our sessions, however, for the babies seem to enjoy the special time that has been set aside for them and their peers.

   At home, your intuition will guide you in flowing with your baby's cycle of attention.

If you are beginning this program with an infant less than a month old, he or she obviously will not want to do all the exercises at once. Some babies don't care for some of the exercises at first, and too many repetitions and changes can be taxing. So begin with just a few exercises, depending on your baby's development and interest. Babies change so much from week to week, and they quickly mature and take great delight in expanding their repertoire of movement and positions.

2. *Move Baby slowly in the first three months to allow for Baby's lack of head control, particularly when changing position.*

3. *When necessary, exercise without Baby in order to continue working on your recovery* (if she is fussy, for instance, asleep, or visiting elsewhere). You may want to continue a prenatal exercise program, such as that presented in *Marie Osmond's Exercises for Mothers-to-Be.* Or try the exercises without Baby.

4. *Always do the warm-ups.* If you don't have time for the whole program, choose those exercises that meet your needs, your baby's interest, and time permit, but always begin with warm-ups, slow down gradually before stopping, and rest and relax afterward if Baby allows.

5. *Always move slowly and coordinate your breathing with the exercises.* Inhale as you pause. Exhale as you exert or stretch. But do not push yourself. Avoid fatigue and that feeling in your muscles known as the "burn." (The "burn" is simply the build-up of waste products from muscle activity that cannot be adequately transported away by the bloodstream.) With practice, you will find you can do more without feeling tired. Just allow yourself to breathe naturally.

   Breath-holding disturbs the harmony between your mind and body, and is easily avoided if you talk or sing to your baby while you exercise.

   All the movements should be done slowly and mindfully, so you can feel what is happening in your whole body. There is no sense in strengthening one muscle group at the expense of another. For example, if doing curl-ups puts a strain on your pelvic floor muscles, even as you exhale, then you should work more on your pelvic floor alone and postpone curl-ups for a few days.

6. *Avoid either raising both legs straight up from the floor when lying on your back or doing full sit-ups.* Both movements can obscure abdominal muscle weakness as the strong thigh muscles do all the work, pulling on your lower spine. These two common exercises are mistakenly thought to strengthen the abdominal muscles, but actually can strain the abdominals and cause back pain. It is more effective to curl-up only half way, and to *lower* your legs (never beyond a 45 degree angle) instead of raising them, in order to engage the abdominal muscles.

7. *Avoid jerking or straining.* It means that a movement or position is too difficult for you and you have to "cheat" by using momentum to do the exercise.

8. *Don't bounce, especially when stretching.* Bouncing will actually stimulate the muscle that you are trying to lengthen to shorten instead. This can cause pain later.

9. *Repeat each exercise about five times in sequence,* but do not push yourself any harder than is comfortable for you. Relaxation is more important than repetitions.

10. *Add progressions for variety.* Multiple repetitions of an exercise can become tiring and boring for both Mother and Baby. Exercises are better if progressed in difficulty. This means that you change the position of your body in order to make the exercise more challenging for a particular muscle group. Specific progressions are suggested for many of the exercises. Progressions are listed in sequence.

11. *It is a good idea to begin walking, swimming, dancing, cycling, or whatever aerobic activity appeals to you as soon as you feel ready.* This gentle mother and baby program is an ideal preparation for more vigorous exercises. Most new mothers soon find that they need to have time for themselves away from Baby, and to work out at a more advanced pace. Going outside the home, either outdoors for jogging (if the pelvic floor has fully recovered) or to a dance or exercise group for some stronger physical exercise, will achieve both aims.

12. *Be ready to move on.* Although you can continue to exercise with your child, and have fun together in water and with the balls, Baby will wriggle out of most of these activities when he or she starts to crawl. At that time, Baby will want to do more independent exploration of his world and he will have developed excellent motor abilities.

   It is part of the bittersweet joy of parenting that we have to let go of one stage and move into the next, which will also have its delights and challenges. Life is growth and change, and nobody can teach us that as well as our children.

4
Warm-ups

Warm-ups are simple movements that gently increase your circulation and prepare your joints and muscles for activity to prevent tissue strain or injury. Try to breathe normally throughout. Be aware of your whole body at all times, making sure, for example, that your shoulders are not tensing up toward your ears, or your lower back hollowing, or your feet rolling inward.

These exercises are done sitting in the "tailor position." Make sure that you alternate the position of your ankles, to give equal stretch to each of your thigh muscles. Baby does not actively participate in the warm-ups, but will enjoy watching your movements. Exercises One, Two, and Three can actually be done in any upright position, each time you hold or nurse your baby.

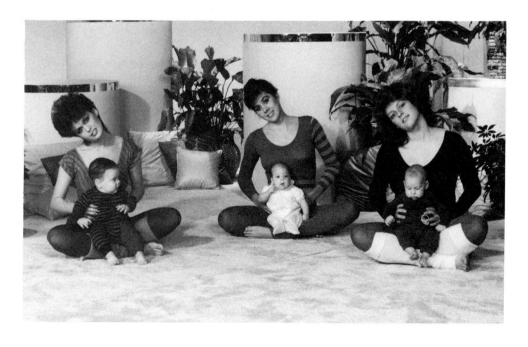

ONE: *Head and Neck Stretches*

Your head and neck is the starting point for warming-up into exercising. You probably have noticed that your neck and upper shoulders are tense and tired from lifting and carrying your baby. These stretches help relieve that tension.

STARTING POSITION

Sit like a tailor, with your knees bent, thighs apart, and ankles crossed or beside each other. Baby can rest in your lap. Keep your shoulders down from your ears.

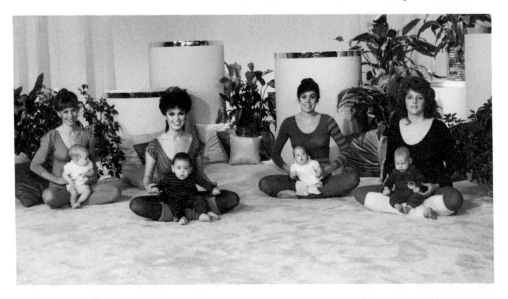

"Stretching my neck feels so good, because most of the time I'm hunched forward over the baby."

1. Let your head drop all the way forward, hanging with its own weight. Slowly lift it up and let it drop forward again.

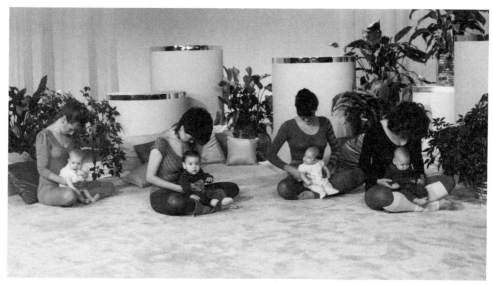

2. Face forward, and stretch your head from side to side, as if to bring your ear toward your shoulder.

You can combine these movements into head rolls if they feel comfortable.

COMMON ERROR

• Raising your shoulder to your ear, which tenses your neck and shoulders.

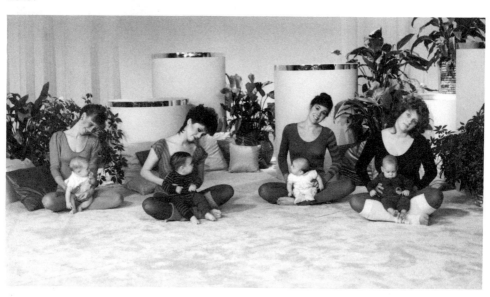

TWO: **Elbow Circles**

This movement stretches and mobilizes your shoulders and strengthens the muscles between your shoulder blades.

STARTING POSITION

Sit in the tailor position with Baby in your lap. Rest your fingertips on your shoulders.

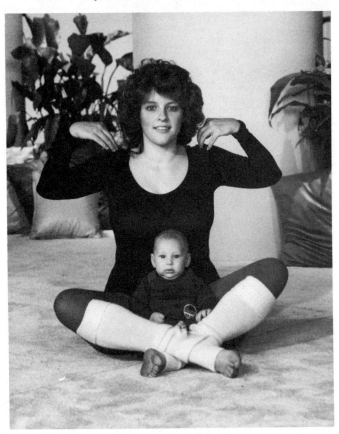

Circle your arms up, back, and down, imagining a piece of chalk on each elbow drawing larger and larger circles. Touch your elbows in front and keep them touching all the way up to eye level if you can. Always move your arms in a backward direction—new mothers do not need any more practice in rounding their shoulders since they do this all day long. (If you are nursing while doing this exercise, just move your free arm.)

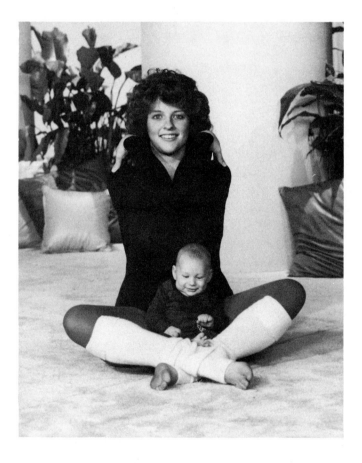

COMMON ERROR

- Circling forward instead of backward.

THREE: Shoulder Circles

Stretching the muscles of your shoulders helps to release tension there which spreads to your neck.

STARTING POSITION

Sit in the tailor position, with Baby in your lap. Stretch your neck tall.

1. Pull one shoulder back and down, and then the other.

2. Move your shoulders back and down together.

COMMON ERROR

• Raising your shoulders toward your ears, instead of emphasizing the downward stretch.

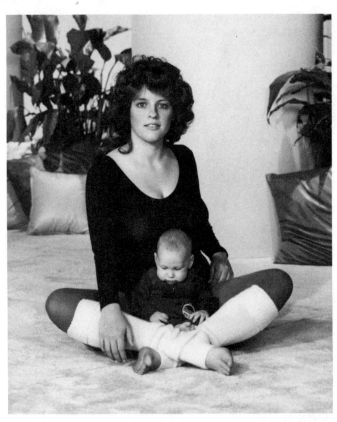

*"Just a few shoulder circles help to make
me feel more comfortable right away."*

FOUR: **Backward Arm Stretch**

This exercise helps improve your posture by stretching the front of your chest and shoulders, and stimulates circulation to your chest and breasts. Holding this stretch will strengthen the muscles of your upper back and your shoulder blades.

STARTING POSITION

Sit in the tailor position, with Baby in your lap. Clasp your hands behind your back.

Keep your elbows straight, and raise your arms as high as you can behind your back.

COMMON ERROR

Leaning forward so that it appears that your arms are being raised. Having Baby on your lap, however, helps prevent this!

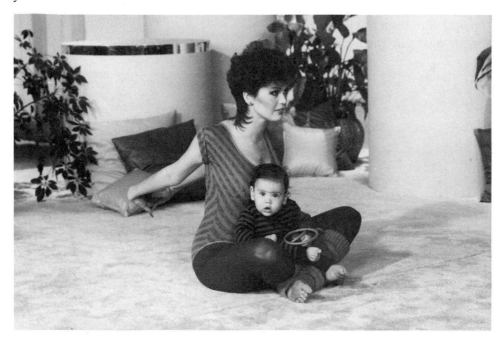

"By the end of the day I have such an upper backache. I love to squeeze my shoulder blades together and stretch out that tension."

FIVE: **Spinal Twist**

Stretching and twisting your spine will relieve stiffness and aching from all the forward-bending that is necessary in the day of a new mother. This exercise keeps the small, deep muscles around your spine supple and enhances their blood circulation.

STARTING POSITION
Tailor sitting, with Baby in your lap. Place your left hand on your right knee.

1. Stretch your spine tall, and twist your trunk to the right. Place your right hand on the floor close to your buttocks. Use your arms to ease you further into the twist. Exhale as you stretch, hold the pose, and stretch a little more on your next outward breath.

2. Repeat to the other side, making sure you always stretch tall in the center position before turning.

COMMON ERRORS
- Allowing your opposite buttock to come off the floor. One point must remain fixed for stretching to occur.

- Twisting with a slouched back.

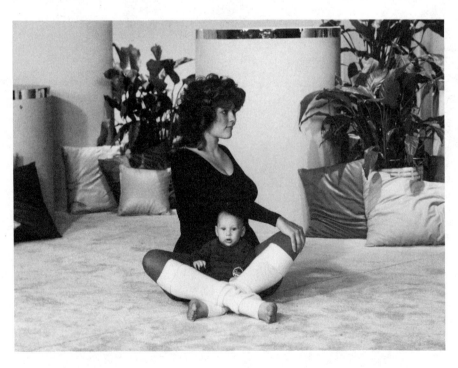

5

Exercising
As You Sit

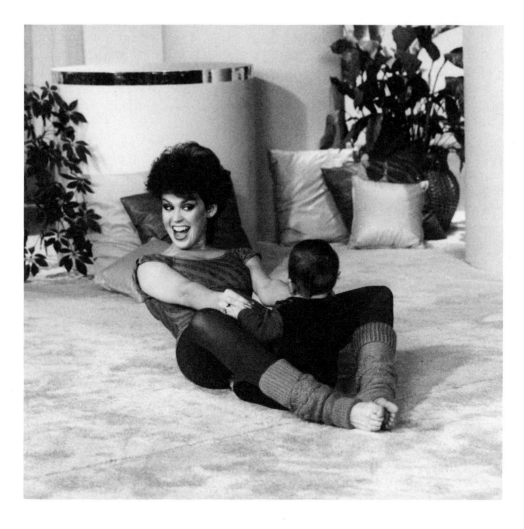

ONE: *Pelvic Floor Contractions*

The pelvic floor muscles, which we discussed in Chapter 1, are hidden deep in the pelvis, and their strength and control is essential to your health and comfort.

Basically, there is just one movement you can make with these muscles—a squeezing and drawing-up of your three inside passages, the urethra, vagina, and anus. You use these important muscles when you interrupt your urine flow (a good check of your muscle strength) and when you squeeze your partner's penis during intercourse.

Pelvic floor exercises can be done any place, any time, and in any position. Try to practice these exercises in positions where your legs are open, so that you are not confused by the more powerful activity in your inner thigh or buttock muscles. It is more difficult, but nevertheless necessary, to exercise your pelvic floor in standing and squatting, where gravity adds to the load of your internal organs.

You should do at least fifty pelvic floor contractions a day, for the rest of your life. However, the pelvic floor muscles tire easily, so just do three or four contractions in a series and rest for a couple of minutes before repeating. Intersperse pelvic floor contractions throughout your exercise program—do a few each time you pause or rest. You can also incorporate them into your daily routine—try to remember to do a few each time you go to the bathroom, come to a stop light, or pick up your baby.

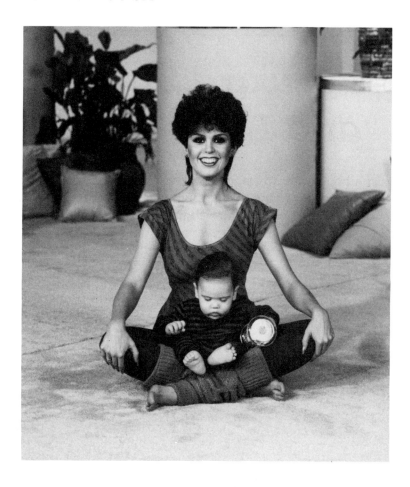

STARTING POSITION

Tailor sitting, with Baby in your lap. Tighten your pelvic floor muscles, with special emphasis on the vaginal area. See if you can feel the muscle contracting deep inside, about the middle third of your vagina. Tighten to a count of three, hold for a count of three, and relax to a count of three.

PROGRESSION

Increase the time intervals to a count of four, and then five. Don't try to hold your pelvic floor tight for more than ten seconds, or to do more than about five contractions in a row.

COMMON ERRORS

• Many women have difficulty even identifying their pelvic floor muscles, particularly if they have not exercised this area of their body prior to childbirth. When a muscle is weak, the body will always try to compensate with a neighboring muscle, and women often squeeze their thighs or buttocks instead of the inside pelvic muscles.

• Holding the breath and bearing down, instead of exhaling and pulling up the muscular hammock.

TWO: **Forward Stretch and Lean-back**

This is a combination exercise for you and your baby. Stretching forward relieves tightness in your hips, inner thighs, and lower back. Leaning back and curling forward exercises your abdominal muscles. Baby will enjoy watching you and joining in with your movements.

Always pull Baby up slowly. Very young babies will need support at the shoulders as they have less head control. Older babies need only to be held by the hands and may pull themselves into a standing position during this exercise.

STARTING POSITION

Sit with your knees apart and the soles of your feet together, with Baby lying on his or her back, between your legs, using your feet as a pillow.

1. Stretch forward to kiss your baby. Breathe out as you stretch.

2. Hold your baby's arms and gently assist him or her to come up to a sitting position, while you slowly lean backward. Inhale as you sit up, exhale as you lean back. Round and lower your back until your abdominal muscles start to tremble—but do not go all the way to the floor.

COMMON ERROR

• Bouncing forward, instead of stretching slowly. Bouncing causes muscles to tighten instead of lengthen and can injure tendons.

*"This is my baby's favorite exercise
because he's always trying
to pull himself up."*

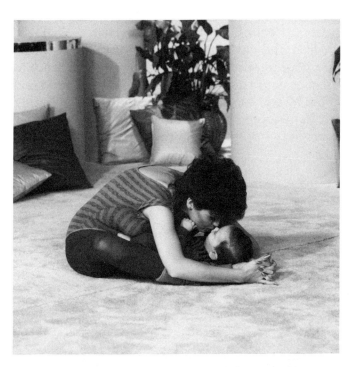

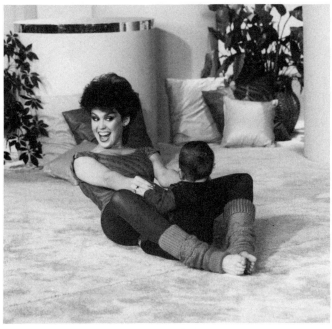

THREE: **Ankle Rides**

This movement is great fun for your baby, and the baby acts as a weight on your ankle, which will firm and strengthen your front thigh muscles. This position is also good for your hip flexibility and you need to have a slim abdomen so that you can bring your thighs close to your chest. It is a real challenge to keep your spine straight in this position. Fully straightening your knee will stretch your hamstrings.

If you want to take the easy way out, this exercise can be done in a chair.

STARTING POSITION

Sit with your knees bent and your legs crossed so that your right thigh rests on your left thigh. Both your feet must be flat on the floor. Make sure that you are sitting on your "sit bones" and that your spine is straight. Sit Baby on your right ankle or lie a smaller baby on her front along your shin. Hold Baby's hands.

Raise your right foot until the knee is straight, taking your baby up for a ride, and then lower it to the floor. After a few repetitions, change legs.

COMMON ERROR

• Often Mother loses the starting position and slouches forward, lifting her whole leg from the hip instead of just the knee. This incorrect movement is very tiring and does not focus on the thigh muscles.

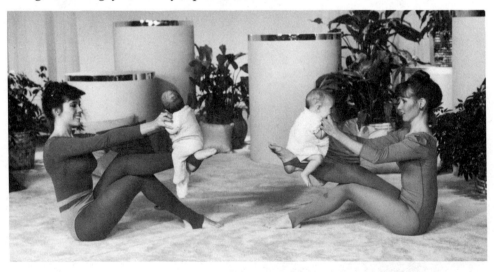

"Lifting the baby is hard work for my thighs, and they certainly need it!"

6

Exercising on Your Back

After childbirth, your abdominal muscles will be loose and stretched. Postpartum women are generally dismayed and discouraged by the appearance and function of their abdominal muscles and want to work them back into shape as soon as possible. The most effective way to do this is lying on your back so that the abdominals must work against gravity. Keep in mind, however, that the stretched muscles must be shortened before they can be strengthened.

You need to be patient with the preliminary work of simply returning your stretched abdominal muscles back to their original length before doing progressive strengthening exercises. Don't rush into the exercise progressions, or you risk doing the exercises incorrectly and further straining your weakened abdominal muscles instead of rebuilding them.

Before you do any abdominal exercises on your back, you must check the condition of your abdominal wall. As we saw on page 16 the outmost layer of muscles, the recti, are prone to separation at the midline during pregnancy and birth. It is important to check if your recti muscles have separated, and if so, to work them back together with the special corrective exercise below before doing any curl-ups, or leg rides (which involve leg-lowering movements). You can easily check for separation yourself by doing the exercises on pages 46–47.

Check for Separation of Abdominal Muscles

STARTING POSITION

Lie on your back, knees bent. Keep your shoulders on the floor.

As you exhale, raise your head and shoulders and press your fingers in the "center seam" of your abdomen, above and below your navel. See how many fingers you can insert horizontally into the space between your recti muscles.

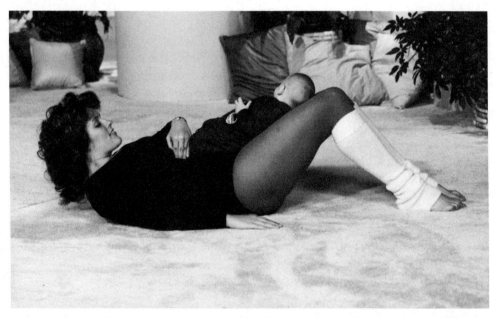

NOTE: *Everyone has a gap of about an inch. If the separation between your recti muscles is less than three fingers' breadth, you and Baby can begin the exercises in this chapter right away. However, if you can fit three or more fingers into the gap, you will need to do the corrective exercise below to close the gap before progressing to curl-ups and leg-lowering exercises. (Other abdominal exercises, such as on all-fours, are fine.)*

Modified Head Raises for Separated Abdominal Muscles

STARTING POSITION

Lie on your back, knees bent. Cross your hands over your waist so that one wrist is above the other.

As you exhale, raise your head, and draw your abdominal muscles together with your hands. Keep your shoulders on the floor.

COMMON ERRORS

- Placing the hands too far apart.
- Exhaling too quickly and allowing the abdominal wall to bulge.
- Bringing the shoulders off the floor, which will increase the gap, as those deeper abdominal muscles insert into the center seam.

NOTE: *Do a few of these head raises half a dozen times throughout the day until you can fit only one or two fingers into the gap when your head is raised. Then begin doing curl-ups, but keep observing and checking the gap in case you progress too fast and the muscles start to open up again.*

ONE: *Head Raises*

This is a warm-up exercise for the abdominal muscles, and the emphasis you place on exhalation promotes fuller breathing. Your abdominal muscles move in toward your spine on outward breath, and frequent abdominal wall tightening helps to shorten the stretched muscles and tone the skin. This exercise is the same as the preceding one, except that you're not supporting your recti muscles with your hands. It will also help the recti muscles regain their tone and normal position (as long as your shoulders don't leave the floor).

Placing your baby in this position encourages his head-raising ability. Gentle blowing when you exhale stimulates Baby's attention, or you can talk to him or imitate his sounds to stimulate his speech.

STARTING POSITION
Lie on the floor, knees bent, with Baby lying face-down on your chest.

Inhale first, and as you exhale, raise your head, blowing onto Baby's face and pulling in your abdominal muscles as hard as you can. Visualize your belly button approaching your backbone. When you have breathed out all your air, relax your head back to the floor and repeat.

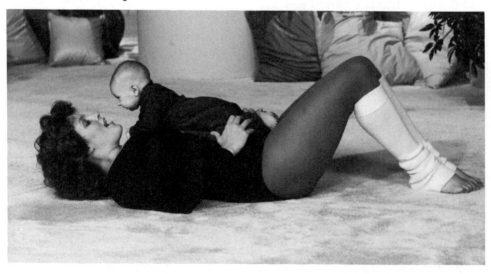

TWO: *Curl-ups (Straight and Diagonal)*

NOTE: *Do not do curl-ups without first checking your abdominal wall. It makes no sense to ask your abdominal muscles to raise your shoulders off the floor if they cannot stay parallel with just the weight of your head.*

Curl-ups, which strengthen your straight and diagonal abdominal muscles, are one of the more difficult and most important exercises a postpartum mother can do. Baby's attention is engaged watching Mother's movement while resting against her legs.

STARTING POSITION
Lie on the floor, knees bent, with Baby lying against your thighs.

1. Inhale first, and as you exhale, bring your head and shoulders forward off the floor. Curl up just halfway—your waist stays on the floor. Slowly uncurl, relax, and inhale.

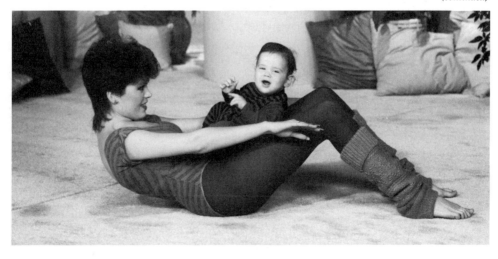

(continued)

"These are the ones to get that tummy flat again."

Curl-ups (continued)

2. Repeat as on page 49, but moving in a diagonal direction—bringing your right shoulder toward your left hip, rolling back, resting, and then rolling your left shoulder toward your right hip.

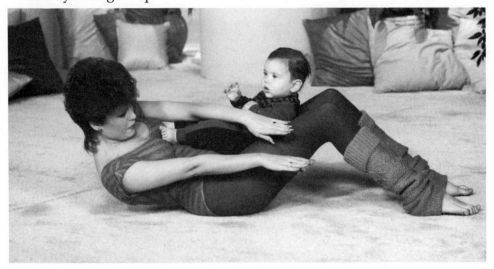

PROGRESSIONS

▲ Repeat the exercise in all three directions with your arms folded across your chest. This position is more difficult because your arms do not help to bring you forward.

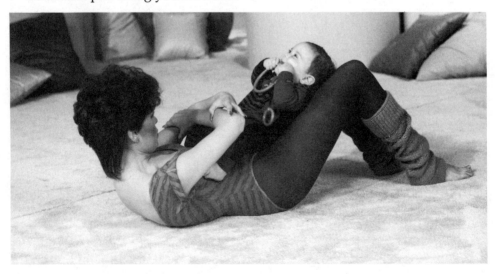

▲ Repeat with your hands clasped behind your head, or at the side of your head. This increases the length of the load that your abdominals must raise.

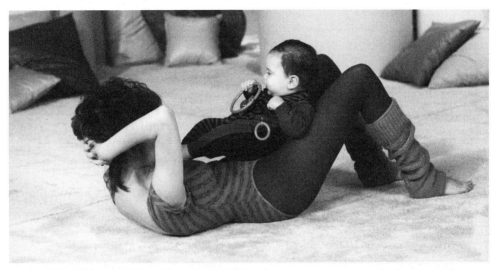

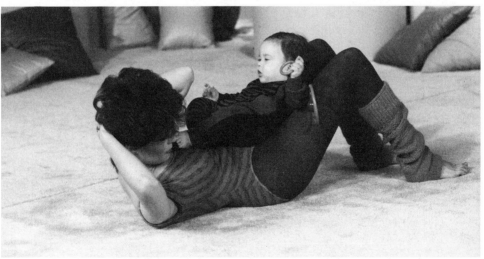

"This is a hard exercise, but it's wonderful fun playing peek-a-boo with Stephen."

THREE: **Bridging**

Raising your hips off the floor strengthens the muscles of your buttocks and back. Your baby acts as a weight to make the exercise more challenging. Baby enjoys riding up and down and sideways. If you give just minimal support, Baby will have to work with his or her trunk muscles to maintain balance.

STARTING POSITION

Lie on your back, knees bent, with Baby lying back against your thighs or sitting on your pelvis. Have your feet at a comfortable distance away from your buttocks. Hold onto Baby's hands or place your hands on Baby's hips.

Tilt your pelvis to flatten your lower back. Keep your pelvis tilted back and slowly raise your hips off the floor to make a "bridge." Lift up slowly, vertebra by vertebra, and keep breathing throughout.

PROGRESSIONS

▲ Place your feet further away from your buttocks. This makes your buttocks work harder to raise your pelvis.
▲ Drop one hip, and then the other while your hips are raised. Return and repeat.

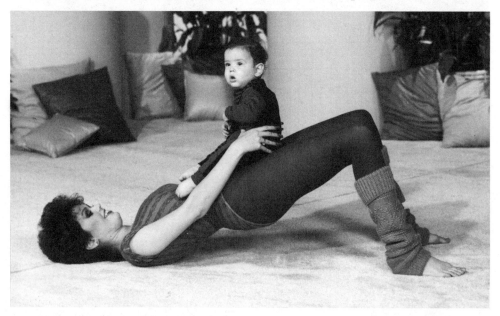

"Stephen loves these rides, and they're great for his balance."

FOUR: *Baby Lifts*

This exercise strengthens your elbows and shoulders for carrying your baby. Baby's neck and back muscles are stimulated and he or she enjoys the vertical movement through space and being higher than Mother for a change. The raised position encourages Baby to extend his legs and trunk, moving them like the tail of a whale.

STARTING POSITION
Lie on your back, knees bent, with Baby lying face-down on your chest, your hands grasping each side of his trunk midway between his ribs and pelvis.

Inhale first, then as you exhale, lift Baby up in the air, over your face, straightening your elbows. Hold him up a minute and then bend your elbows and let him rest down on your chest again. You can also bring Baby down for a kiss between lifts.

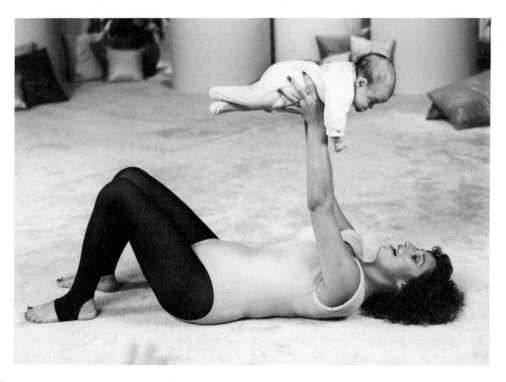

"Babies love to fly! Look how they open their arms and legs."

FIVE: Leg Rides

NOTE: *Do not do this exercise if your abdominal muscles are separated.*

This is one of the most popular exercises in our program. Keeping your lower back flat on the floor during leg movements (with the added weight of Baby) is strong work for your abdominal muscles. Raising your head and shoulders off the floor is also a good abdominal muscle workout. Baby loves the horizontal change of direction and different body position, and his head, back, and arm muscles are stimulated.

STARTING POSITION

Lie on your back, knees bent over your waist, feet off the floor, with Baby lying face-down along your shins. Hold onto Baby's hands.

1. Tilt your pelvis to flatten your lower back and gradually lower your legs, attempting to straighten your knees as you approach a 45 degree angle. (You will not be able to straighten them all the way and still hold on to Baby's hands.) Then bring your knees back up over your waist again. The important point is not to allow your lower back to arch off the floor. Keep your head and shoulders on the floor and exhale while you lower your legs.

NOTE: *Do not lower your legs beyond a 45 degree angle. When your legs leave or approach the floor together, it is virtually impossible to control your pelvic tilt. Like a seesaw, your lower back will arch off the floor first and you risk straining both your back and your abdominals. Holding onto Baby's hands in the beginning helps to prevent this by limiting the distance your legs can be lowered.*

2. Keep your knees over your waist and now curl up to kiss your baby. Then roll back to rest your head and shoulders on the floor and lower your knees again.

PROGRESSION

As your baby gets older and grasps your legs, it will not be necessary to hold his or her hands and you can work on lowering your legs so that your knees become completely straight at a 45 degree angle. If you can do this, keeping your back in contact with the floor, you have 100 percent abdominal muscle strength.

COMMON ERRORS

- Straightening the knees too soon so that the baby tends to slide off. This creates too long a lever to lower from that height.
- Not keeping your lower back on the floor as your knees move away. Using your abdominal muscles to maintain your pelvic tilt is the major point of this exercise.
- Holding your breath instead of exhaling during the exertion.

''This exercise really works on my abdominal muscles,
especially as Stephen is growing so big
. . . he's quite a weight.''

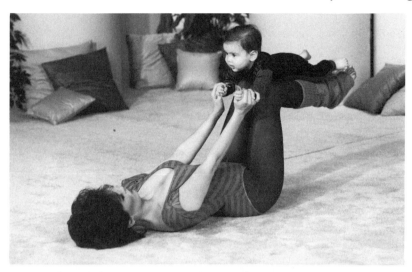

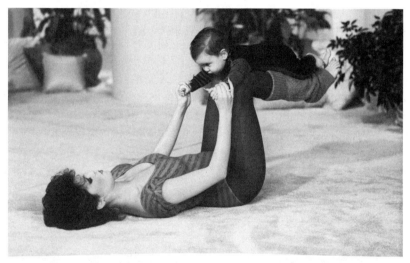

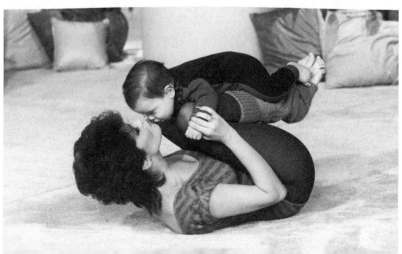

7

Exercising on Your Hands and Knees

In the hands-and-knees exercises, Baby does not engage in direct movement, but remains in close visual contact with you. Baby will enjoy following your arm and head movements, especially if you have long hair.

Movements in the all-fours position need special attention because you cannot use vision as you are accustomed to doing in other positions, but instead you must develop your joint and muscle sense. Exercises in this position help to relieve backache. If you do these exercises in your underwear or a leotard, you can clearly see the state of your abdominal wall.

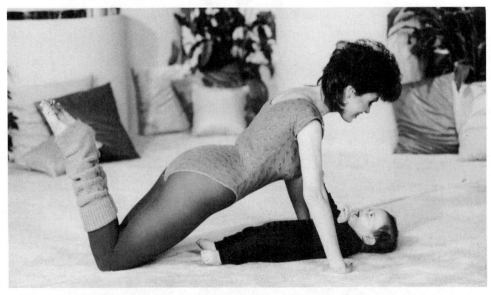

ONE: *Pelvic Tilts*

Tilting your pelvis upward is achieved by pulling in your abdominals and tucking under your buttocks. It is a subtle movement that you want to emphasize in the lower part of your spine rather than in the upper part, as in the common "angry cat" exercise. Most women are already too rounded in their upper backs, and too hollowed in their lower backs. On your hands and knees, your abdominals must work against gravity to raise your pelvis.

STARTING POSITION

Get on all fours, with your hands under your shoulders, knees under your hips. Baby lies on his back facing you.

(continued)

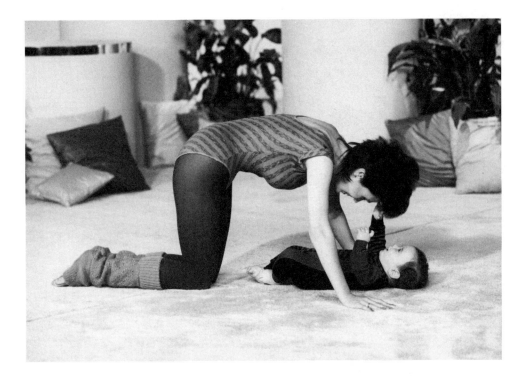

"In this position I can see what a lot of work my belly needs!"

Pelvic Tilts (continued)

As you exhale, raise your pelvis to round your lower back. Relax back to a neutral position when you inhale. As a general rule, don't let your lower back sag down unless your spine is flat there.

COMMON ERROR
- Allowing the spine to hollow more than it is raised.

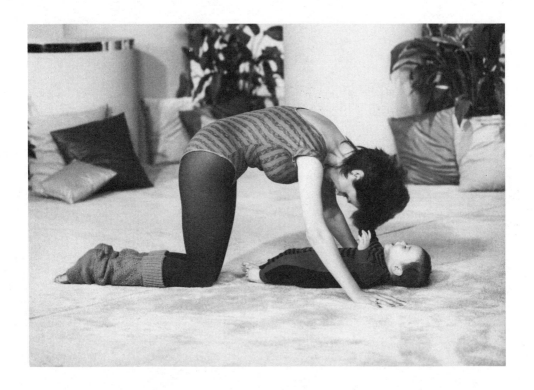

"I can feel this doing my back good!"

TWO: **Side Bends**

Side-bending while maintaining a pelvic tilt works your front (i.e., underneath) abdominals as well as those at your side. This exercise will help you to regain your waistline. Baby will often track your arc of movement with her eyes.

STARTING POSITION

Get on all fours, hands under your shoulders, knees under your hips. Baby lies on her back, facing you.

Raise your pelvis, keep your back as flat as a table top, and bend from left to right to look at your buttocks. Exhale as you bend, inhale when you return to the center position.

COMMON ERROR

• Allowing the spine to hollow while you side bend.

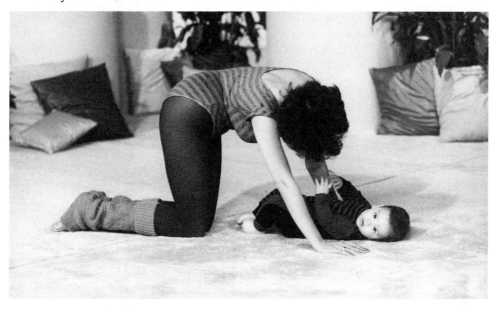

"This week he has really started to follow my head movements."

THREE: *Push-ups*

This movement strengthens your arms and shoulders, which will make it easier for you to lift and carry your baby. With your hands turned in and fingertips facing each other, you will better develop the triceps muscles which extend your elbows.

STARTING POSITION

Get on all fours, hands under your shoulders, knees under your hips. Baby lies on the floor, facing you.

1. Raise your feet off the floor, tilt your pelvis back, bend your elbows, and lower your body to kiss your baby. Keep your shoulders, hips, and knees aligned.

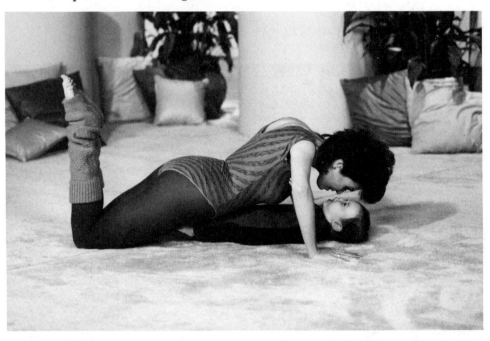

"Doing this one right is a real challenge
. . . my baby thinks it's a lot of fun!"

2. Inhale, and as you exhale,
straighten your elbows. Make
your arms and abdominals do the
work. Between the movements,
for variety, you can sit back on
your heels, stretching your arms
and back, and kiss Baby's toes.

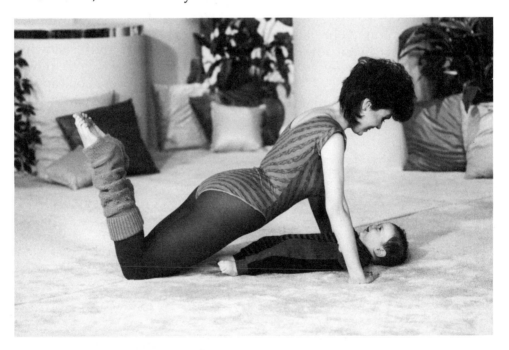

COMMON ERROR

• Lowering just your chest and not
your pelvis, leaving your buttocks
in the air.

FOUR: Alternate Arm and Leg Stretches

These stretches are also progressions of pelvic tilting, for you *must* maintain a correct pelvic tilt while raising and lowering your limbs. Your abdominal muscles raise your pelvis and lower back, which becomes more difficult when your balance is further challenged with alternate arm and leg movements. Your balance and coordination will improve with this exercise while you strengthen your abdominals and the muscles of your back, buttocks, shoulders, arms, and legs.

STARTING POSITION

Get on all fours, hands under your shoulders, knees under your hips. Baby rests on the floor, facing you. Position your body so that when you stretch out an arm, your hand is over Baby's chest in his line of vision.

1. Raise your pelvis so that your lower back is flat. Keeping your spine straight and breathing normally, stretch out one arm and engage Baby's attention with your hand. You can wiggle your fingers, or hold a rattle or bright object as you move your arm slowly back and forth, allowing your baby to track your movements with his eyes. You can also tickle Baby's tummy, which stimulates his abdominal muscles. Change arms.

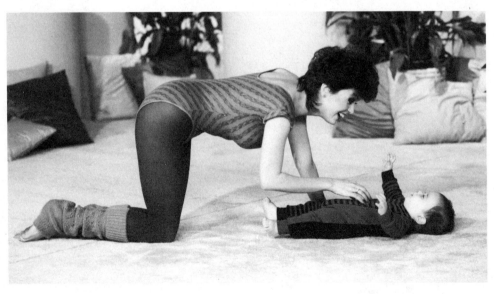

"I do this one with colored ribbons in my hand and he's just fascinated."

2. Hold your spine straight while you bend one knee up toward your nose and then extend it behind you, straightening your leg.

Keep your outstretched leg in line with your body—no higher and no lower than your trunk. Change legs.

(continued)

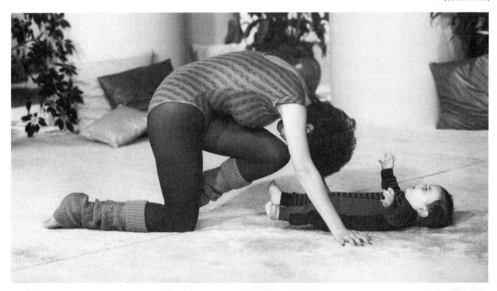

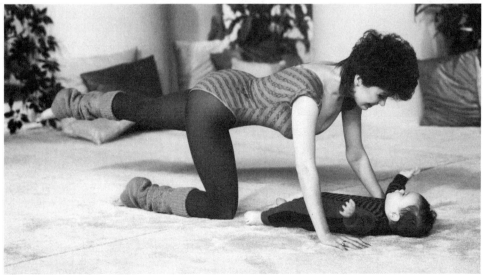

Alternate Arm and Leg Stretches (continued)

PROGRESSION

Now try a combination of opposite arm and leg. Keep your back flat and breathe normally throughout. Flex and extend one leg and stretch out the opposite arm. Develop your body sense, and visualize your whole body aligned—arm, back, leg. S-t-r-e-t-c-h as you hold this position. Continue to stimulate your baby's visual tracking with your hand while you keep your balance. Change sides.

COMMON ERRORS

- Allowing your back to hollow, especially by raising your leg too high, which also twists the hip.
- Raising the arm and leg on the same side, which is an unstable position.

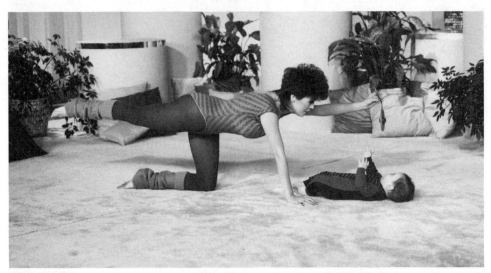

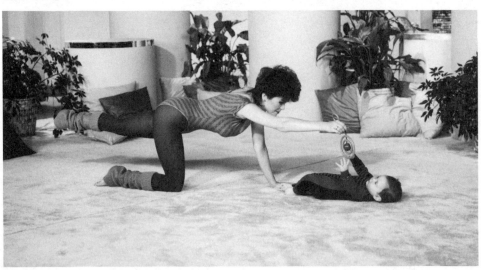

8
Exercising While You Stand

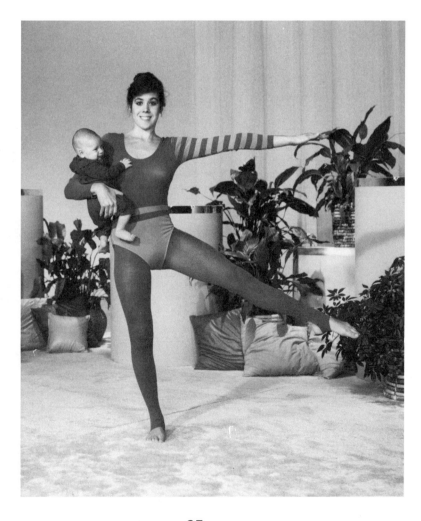

ONE: *Baby Swings*

This exercise is always popular with babies. They love the stimulation of being moved back and forth through space, which encourages them to hold up their head and extend their legs. Mothers strengthen their arms and shoulders while mobilizing their spines.

STARTING POSITION

Stand with your feet apart, holding Baby in a face-down position at your waist level, with your hands under his belly.

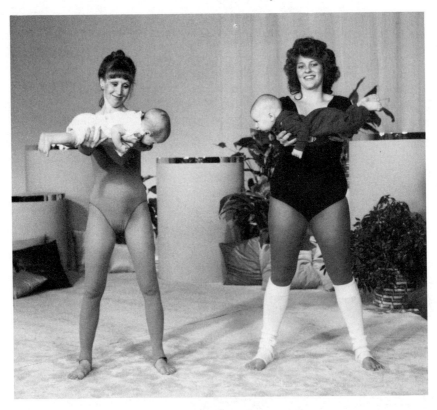

"He doesn't like lying on his front yet, but when I swing him in the air like this he thinks it's great!"

Stretch out your arms and turn your body from side to side, moving Baby like an airplane.

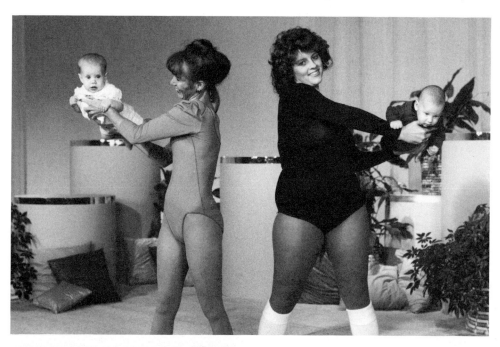

PROGRESSION

Hold your arms higher—shoulder height is more difficult than waist level.

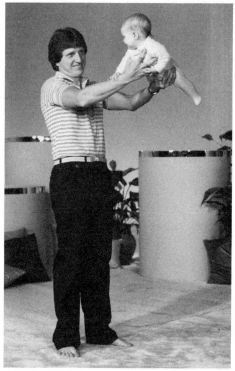

TWO: *Hip-hiking*

In this exercise, the baby acts as a weight on your hip, which provides an extra challenge for your side abdominals. As you work on regaining your waistline, Baby enjoys a rhythmical ride. This exercise is fun to do with another parent and baby—you greet, part, and then meet again.

STARTING POSITION

Stand with your feet apart and Baby astride one hip, facing into your body.

As in belly dancing, raise your pelvis on the side that supports Baby and come up onto the toe of that leg. Raise and lower that hip several times before sitting Baby on your other hip and hiking it.

PROGRESSION

Stand on one leg. Then, taking small steps with your other leg, move around in a circle, hiking up the Baby on your hip with each step. After completing one circle, put Baby astride your other hip and make a circle in the opposite direction.

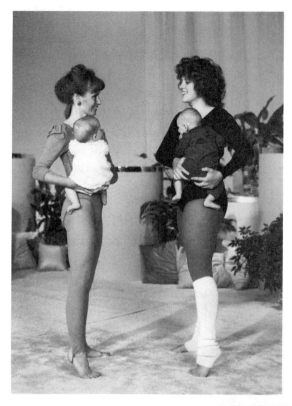

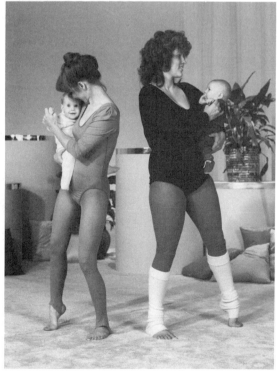

THREE: Leg Swings

This exercise strengthens the muscles of your standing leg as well as the leg that you swing. Most people find it difficult to stand on one leg, especially with the extra weight of holding a baby. (You may want to touch the wall—for balance only, not support—in the beginning.) Baby enjoys watching your leg movements.

STARTING POSITION
Stand with your feet apart, Baby astride one hip.

1. Balance on the leg that supports Baby, and swing your other leg backward and forward.

(continued)

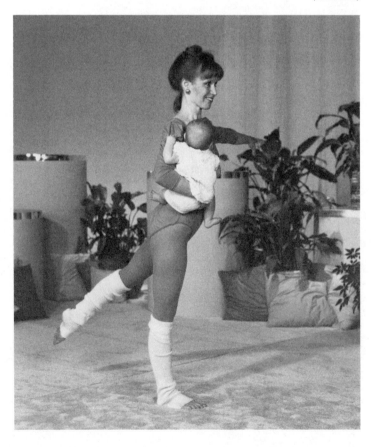

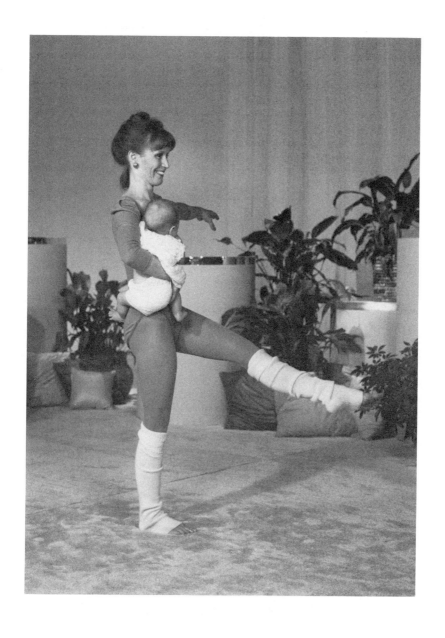

Leg Swings (continued)

2. Now swing your leg out to the side, bring it in front, then out to the side again, and then behind your other leg.

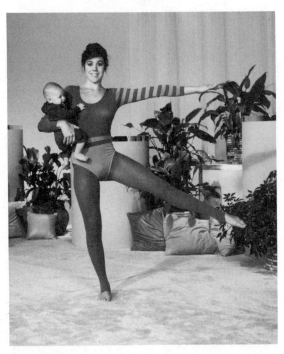

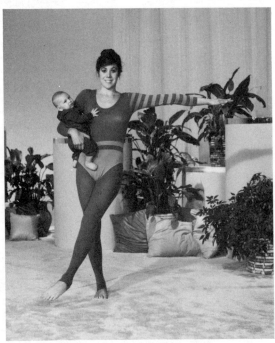

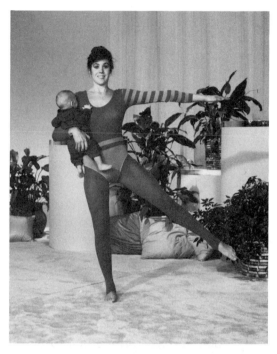

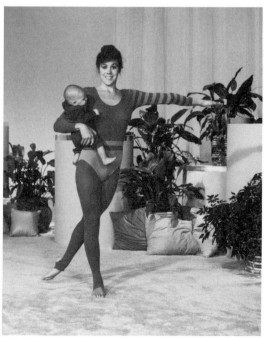

FOUR: Lunge Stretch

This is a difficult position to hold and demands much of your hip, buttock, and leg muscles. Baby explores balance on your thigh. Your ankle mobility and strength will improve.

STARTING POSITION

Stand with your feet wide apart, left foot facing forward and right foot turned out. Sit Baby astride your right thigh, and hold her hands or her hips.

1. Bend your right hip and knee, and lunge to the right. Try to get your right thigh parallel to the floor. (This is a more secure position for Baby, too. If your thigh forms an incline, Baby tends to slide down it!) *Hold* the position and keep breathing—don't bounce. Keep the outer border of your left foot on the floor.

2. To move out of this stretch, "walk" your feet, in and out, in and out, toward the center. When you change sides, lift up Baby from her base and turn your right foot in and your left foot out.

COMMON ERROR

- Bouncing. If you bounce, you will actually stimulate the muscles to tighten instead of allowing them to lengthen.
- Allowing the forward-facing foot to come partially off the floor, which can strain your knee.

*"These exercises seemed easier when I was pregnant. . . .
I sure have a lot of work to do to get back in shape."*

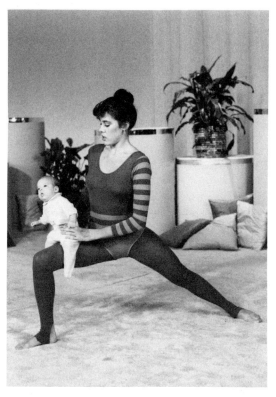

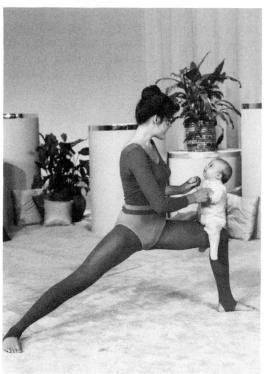

FIVE: Dancing

Babies love movement. It is how they discover themselves and the world. Dancing helps get you back in shape and lets your baby experience spontaneous movement and changes of direction. Try to dance steadily for about fifteen minutes a day with your baby, with whatever style and music is your pleasure.

Carrying the weight of your baby, plus making sure you push off from your toes and lift up your knees, makes the session beneficial for your heart, lungs, and general muscle tone. Remember, you used to run, jump, maybe dance, when Baby was inside you, so Baby need not be treated like a fragile doll.

Try dancing sideways and backward. Hold Baby with outstretched arms as you spin around in a circle. Change your baby's position frequently. Babies love to be held under the belly and will usually lift up their heads and legs. Dance cheek-to-cheek, holding Baby's hand. Older babies enjoy sitting on your shoulders, facing forward and also facing backward.

Spend some time supporting your baby from below so she faces forward and has to use her trunk muscles to stay upright while you move around. Fathers are physically stronger than mothers (and often less tired at the end of the day!) and can continue holding Baby in this position for longer.

If you are exercising with another mother and baby, it is fun to dance together, exchanging babies as described in the next chapter.

9

Exercising with Partners and Mirrors

The following exercises can be done with another parent and child, in groups of several mothers and babies (you may be able to get such a group started in your neighborhood), or simply by using a mirror. They can, of course, be done just by yourself with Baby.

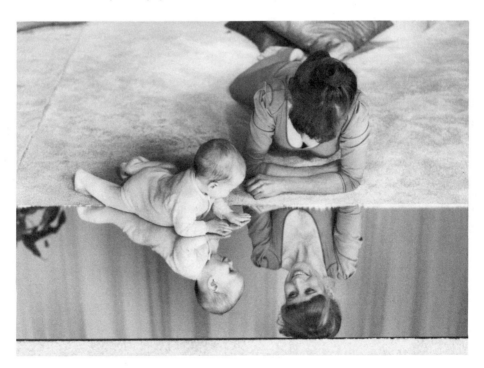

ONE: **Side Bends with Baby**

There are several components to this exercise. Sitting with legs astride and no support behind you is challenging for your back muscles. Spreading your legs and bending your trunk forward stretches your inner thighs and the sides of your torso. Your arm muscles develop as you lift the increasing weight of your baby.

Baby is taken through an 180 degree arc of movement and enjoys the parallel movement of another baby or her own image in a mirror. These movements stimulate the mechanism in Baby's ears which promotes balance.

STARTING POSITION

Partners sit on the floor opposite each other, legs astride and soles of feet touching. Each parent holds her baby by the base so that the babies face each other.

1. Raise and lower the babies in unison. Exhale as you exert!

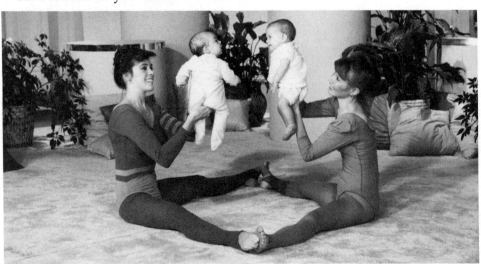

"Look how the babies watch each other!"

2. Now place one hand between Baby's legs and your other hand so it supports the right side of Baby's trunk. (The partner supports his or her baby from the base and on the left side.) Tilt Baby onto his or her right side as you bend sideways, bringing your right ear toward your right knee. Your partner mirrors your movement, moving with his or her baby to their left. Breathe out as you stretch.

3. Return to the center, change hands, and bend with Baby to the other side.

COMMON ERRORS

- Moving the baby from side to side without bending yourself.
- Incorrect positioning of your hands so that Baby is not supported in the direction of the movement.

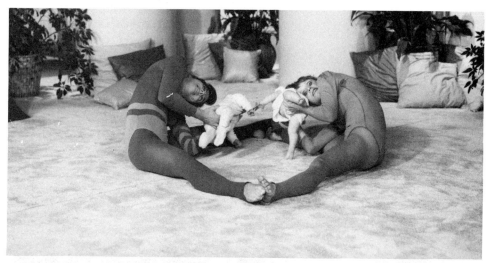

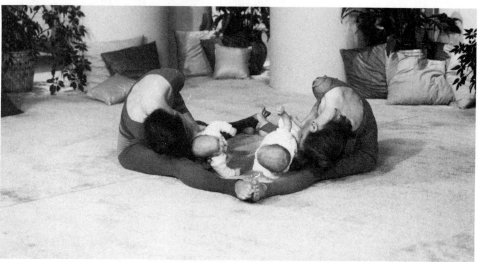

TWO: *Overhead Baby Raises*

This movement builds up power in your arms and shoulders. Your infant's head control and balance will be stimulated. Babies enjoy the surprise of meeting a companion face to face when they are lifted up into the air.

STARTING POSITION

Partners sit back-to-back with their legs crossed or astride. Babies are held by their seats, facing in.

Simultaneously raise both babies up in the air, as you exhale. Lower slowly and inhale.

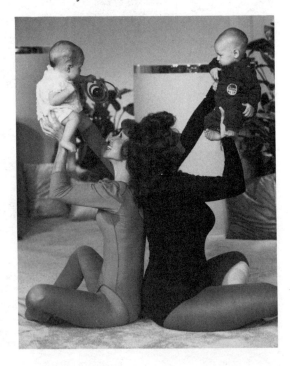

"I wish I'd started this one earlier. My baby is getting so heavy now."

THREE: **Buttock Walk**

This exercise works your abdominals, back, hip, and buttock muscles. The more vigorously you move, the more of a workout your heart and lungs will get as well. Baby enjoys the motion, changes of direction, and interaction with a mirror image or another baby. With minimum support from your hands, Baby's head and trunk control will be challenged.

STARTING POSITION

Sit with your legs outstretched in front of you, your back straight. Make sure you are sitting on your "sit bones" and not slouching. Baby sits side-saddle, or if very small, astride one leg. Place your hands near your baby's hips so that she will need to straighten her back and head for balance.

1. Move forward on your buttocks for a few feet and then move backward. Make sure that you move from your hips, leading with the shoulder on the same side as well. You can move back and forth in a parallel direction with your partner and baby, or in opposite directions so that the babies meet and part and meet again.

2. Face Baby in a different direction, and on your other leg.

3. Exchange babies with your partner so that each parent can enjoy watching her infant's response.

COMMON ERRORS

- Giving baby too much support—i.e., putting your hands under Baby's shoulders, which also restricts her breathing.
- Bending your knees too much instead of moving from your hips.
- Rounding your shoulders.

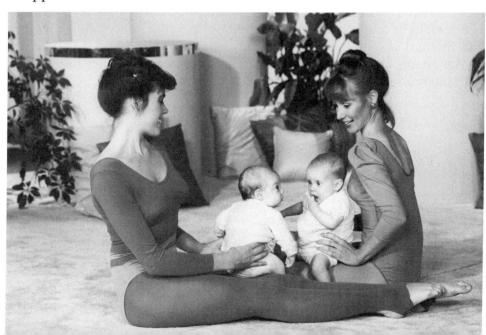

FOUR: *Singing and Dancing*

It's fun to swing the baby inside a blanket, with a partner holding the other end. Baby loves the rhythmical motion. You can sing a nursery song such as "Obediah" while you swing:

Swing me just a little bit higher
Obediah, do;
Swing me just a little bit higher
I love you;
Swing me over the garden wall
But swing me gently so I don't fall;
Just a little higher
Obediah, do!*

Dancing with your baby, with other parents and infants, or with a mirror, is a nice way to vary the exercise activities. You can dance toward and away from the mirror or partner team, turning around in a circle so that babies see each other there one minute, gone the next, and back again. Vary your baby's position frequently, as described in Exercise Five of the last chapter (page 76).

Exchange babies now and then so that you can see all the expressions of delight on your child's face and your baby can look at your responses. (In the early days, parents see more of the top and back of their infant's head, than his face!) It is also fun to feel the different muscle tone and developmental skills of other babies. When you hold an older baby, you'll see what your infant will soon be learning to do with his or her body. If you hold a younger baby, you'll be surprised to realize how much yours has grown, and how hard it is to remember those first weeks.

* This rhyme and other songs are set to music by Pat Carfra, *The Lullaby Lady*, on a cassette tape with an accompanying booklet of words. The tape, and other tapes of children's songs, are available from the Maternal and Child Health Center, 2464 Massachusetts Avenue, Cambridge, MA 02140.

FIVE: **Social Gathering**

Babies become aware of other babies very early, and share a natural affinity with each other. Try putting several babies close together on their fronts or supported in a sitting position. This is lots of fun for parents, too—to watch the puzzlement, smiles, gropes, and other forms of nonverbal communication. Try moving elsewhere in the circle so you can watch your baby's face. This is a good time for a song, or some visual stimulation like blowing bubbles.

Your baby may like to lie face-down on a mirror and see an image of herself. If you get together with other mothers, try placing all the babies around the edge of a mirror. This gives young infants more of a view if they cannot yet hold up their heads for long.

Some babies seem not to like it on their fronts—perhaps they find it too much work to raise and turn their heads. It may help to roll up a towel or blanket to form a support under Baby's chest or to place Baby on a gymnastic ball.

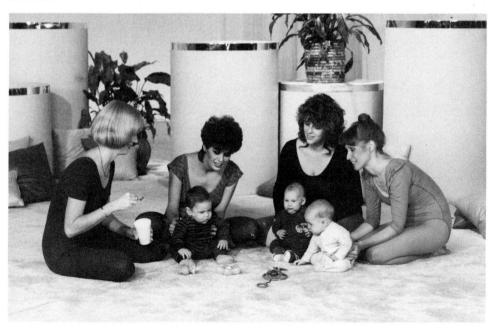

"It's so much fun when the babies start to sit . . . and look at them observing everything so carefully."

SIX: Squat and Stretch

Squatting exercises your thigh muscles and stretches your calves, and it is the most efficient way to lift objects from the floor without straining your back. Baby enjoys a vertical ride and the sharing of this movement with another infant or a mirror image. Movement through space with minimal support challenges Baby's balance and spine control.

STARTING POSITION

Partners stand opposite each other with their feet apart, holding their babies by the base so they face each other.

1. Tilt your pelvis back, bend your knees, and lower yourself and Baby toward the floor. Always squat with your feet flat. (This is a good time to do some pelvic floor contractions.)

2. Slowly lift Baby as you straighten your knees to a standing position, raising Baby over your head. Exhale as you raise the load. Coordinate these movements so they are done simultaneously with your partner's.

3. This exercise is great fun in a group with the mothers forming a circle, running into the center of the room and squatting down with the babies, and then running backward again. Fathers are best at this exercise, with their greater arm strength.

(continued)

*"What would the world do
without babies?"*

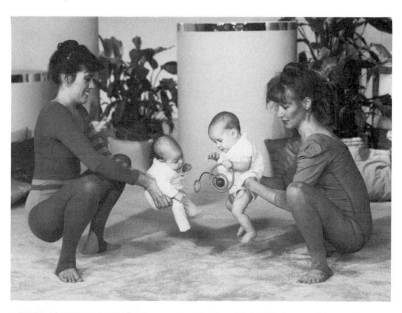

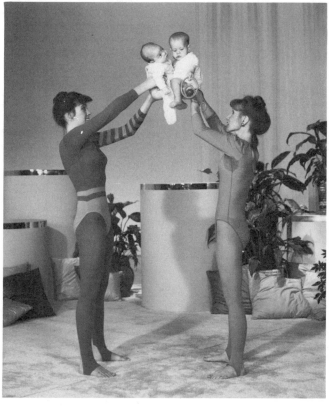

Squat and Stretch (continued)

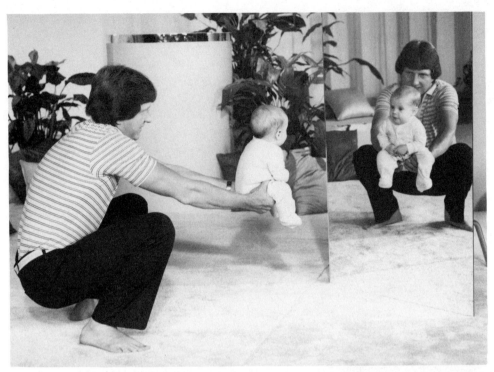

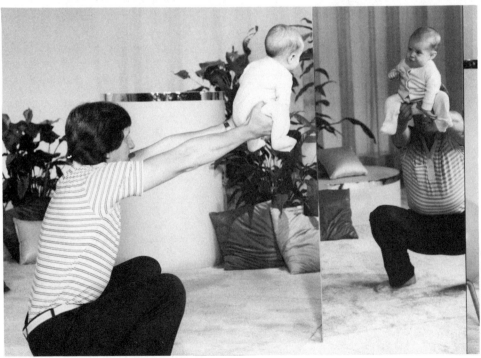

10
Guided Movements for Baby

If you do the following movements regularly with your baby, you will delight in how her response develops each week. You will also enjoy feeling how your baby's body becomes more relaxed.

Baby experiences the range of motion she has at each joint, which is a thrilling exploration of movements she can't yet do well herself. Harmonize with your baby's wishes, gently assisting the limbs as far as they yield. Start gradually, especially with a newborn, and add more movements when the baby seems ready.

Always start with joints that are closer to the body—i.e., loosen the shoulder before the elbow and the elbow before the hand. Move gently, guiding the movement without force or haste, in the spirit of interaction as a form of play, not as a mechanical exercise.

Baby on Her Back

1. Circle Baby's shoulders in an up, out, and down direction. First, do one at a time, then try both together. Baby's elbow can be bent at first, then straightened.

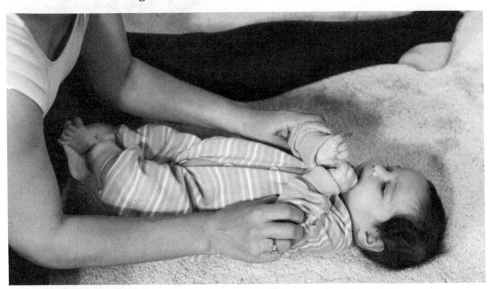

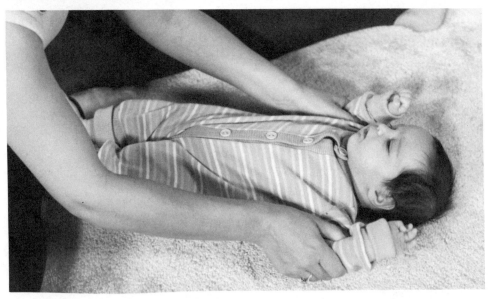

2. Lift one arm up to the ceiling, straightening Baby's elbow, allowing Baby to roll a little. Then bend the elbow all the way back to the floor. Alternate arms.

(continued)

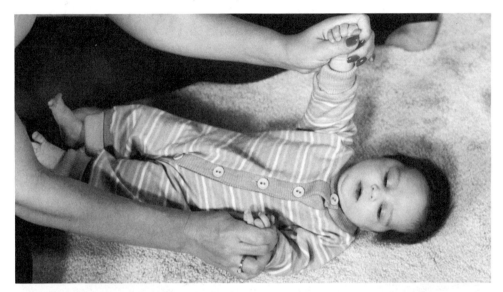

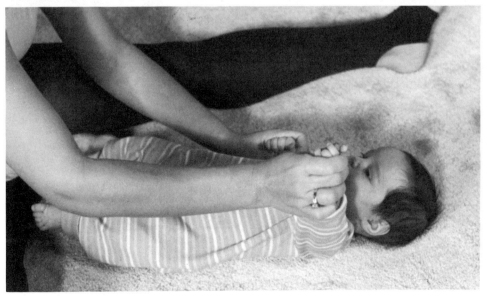

Baby on Her Back (continued)

3. Cross Baby's arms over her chest—opening her arms and then closing them like a hug. Alternate the top arm.

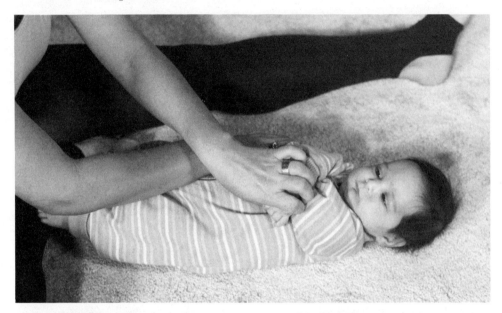

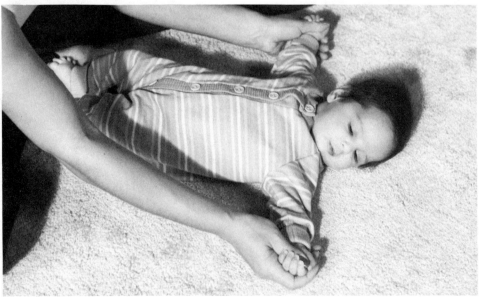

4. Touch Baby's hands to her opposite toe, and alternate.

(continued)

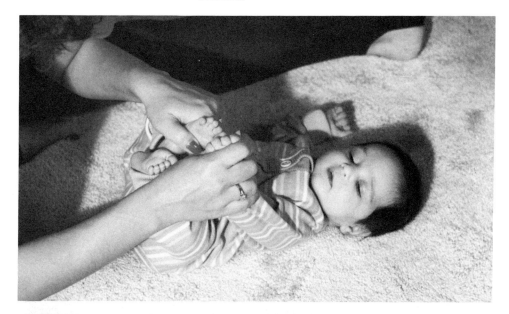

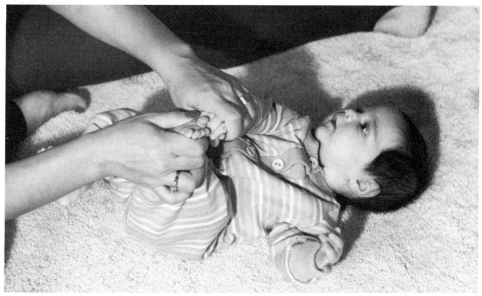

Baby on Her Back (continued)

5. Lifting both legs, rotate Baby's pelvis, first in one direction, then change.

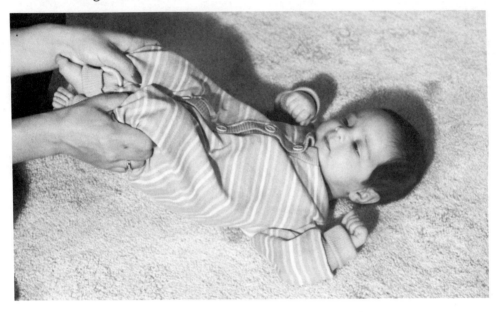

*"Fathers really enjoy doing
these baby exercises!"*

6. Circle each leg up, back, and
down, first separately, then together with the buttocks resting
on the floor.

(continued)

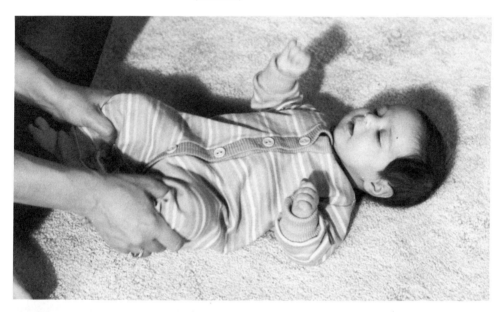

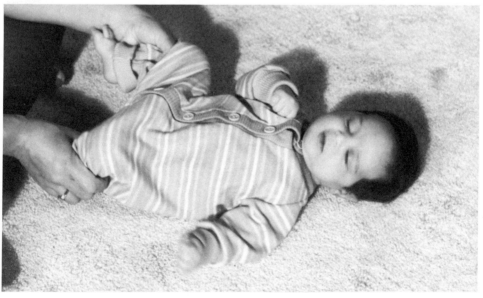

Baby on Her Back (continued)

7. Bend one knee up to Baby's trunk while you straighten her other leg. Alternate legs.

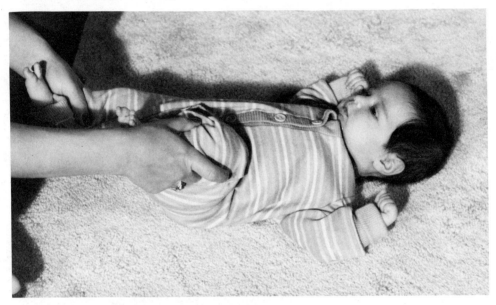

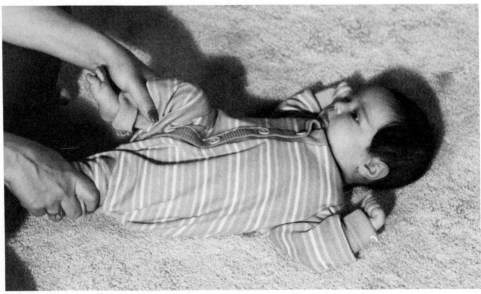

8. Touch the soles of Baby's feet together, and then spread her legs
   sideways.

(continued)

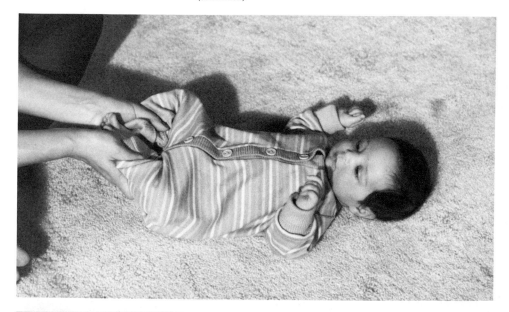

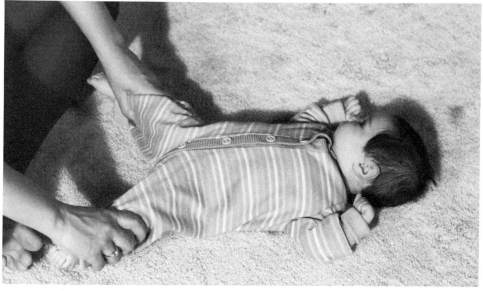

Baby on Her Back (continued)

9. Press gently on Baby's feet—she may kick in response.

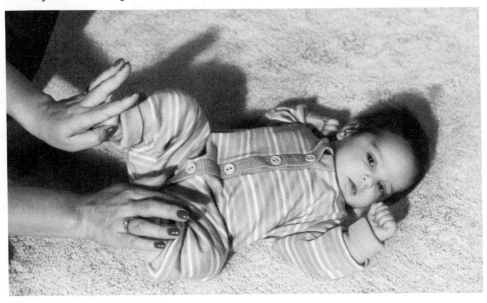

10. Bend up one knee and hip and carefully roll Baby onto her front. Give just minimal assistance—see how much Baby can rotate her own trunk. Circle her toward the side she is facing.

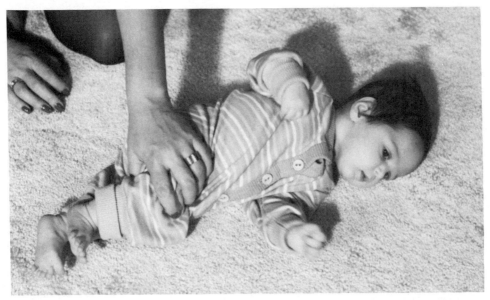

Baby on Her Front

Gently bend one knee under Baby's trunk and alternate, like a crawling movement. With an active baby, if you just press your hands against her feet, she may make this movement automatically. If Baby seems uncomfortable or awkward on her front, you may try forming a wedge under her chest with a small, folded blanket.

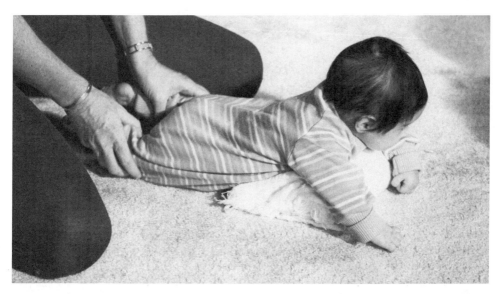

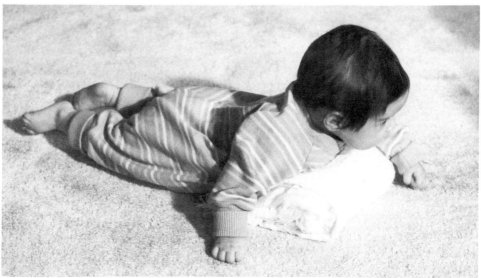

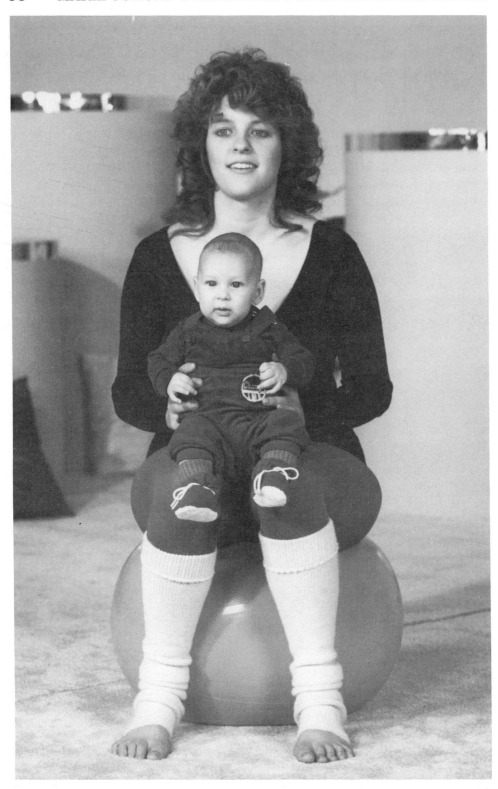

11

Ball Activities

Movement on balls is fun and has benefits for both Mother and Baby. Sitting with a fussy baby on a ball and rhythmically bouncing is a very reliable way to quiet the Baby. Bouncing is a change of sensation for Baby and is less tiring for Mother than standing and rocking. Ball activities will also improve Baby's balance, posture, and righting reactions, and mothers enjoy seeing these skills develop in their babies.

Special exercise balls are available in a small size for infants and toddlers and larger sizes for children and adults. Many mothers at our Center buy the middle size (shown in the photographs), which they can use for their own aerobics, stretching, and strengthening as well as with the baby.* The balls also make handy seats and footrests in the home.

Mostly Baby will be dressed when you play on the ball. However, have Baby undressed, at least sometimes, for ball activities. Skin contact with the ball is ideal, especially for smaller babies who are less secure and experienced. Without clothes, they tend to stick to the surface of the ball and are less likely to slide. Furthermore, Baby enjoys the skin stimulation.

Ball activities are fun to do with partners so babies can roll together and apart.

* Balls can be ordered from the Maternal and Child Health Center, 2464 Massachusetts Avenue, Cambridge, MA 02140.

1. Rest Baby face-down on the ball. Hold her by the buttocks and gently roll her back and forth. When Baby is ready, she will extend her arms, opening her hands, and will straighten her legs. As she gets a little more muscle tone and height, she will enjoy feeling the floor (or your thighs) with her feet on the downward roll and with her hands on the forward roll. As Baby becomes more confident, you can try holding just her ankles and she will outstretch her arms and hands as a protective propping reaction when you go forward.

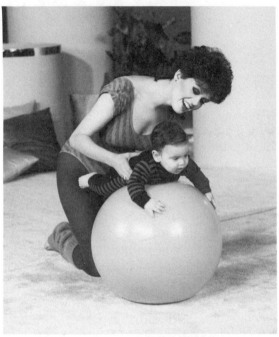

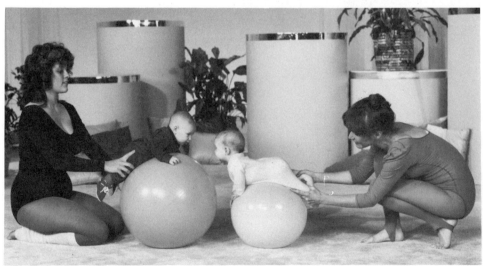

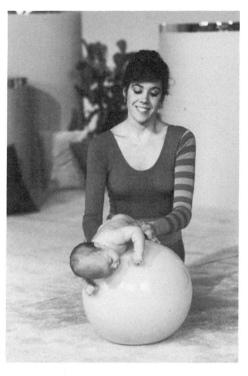

2. Roll the ball from side to side to enhance Baby's righting reactions in this direction.

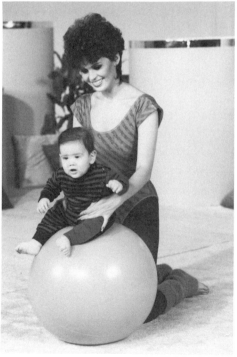

3. When your baby starts to sit, place her in a sitting position on the ball, supporting as little of her trunk as possible. Begin with your hands around her hips, later just holding her thighs. This stimulates your baby's balancing skills as you roll the ball in all directions.

"Best of all, babies like rolling on the ball."

12

Water Games

Baby's first nine months were spent floating in warm fluid, a state of oceanic bliss. Many mothers wonder, then, why their baby doesn't like his bath. Most baby baths only permit a wash—Baby is not free and floating. It is much easier and more enjoyable to have the baby take baths in the regular bathtub with you and/or your partner.

Fill up the tub as high as you can, and your baby will gradually explore movement in water. You'll find you can support just Baby's head and he will joyfully move around. If you are bathing along with the baby in the tub, place a towel on the floor and put the baby on it before you get out. Make sure the room, and if possible the towel, is warm, because air always feels cool to a wet body.

Babies also like showers, but they are more difficult to manage because Baby is so slippery to soap and hold.

Many community centers now offer swimming sessions for mothers and babies. Swimming is also an excellent exercise for Mother to do postpartum, and after having some fun with Baby in the water, you can keep an eye on him beside the pool while you swim some laps. There is much interest today in "drownproofing," or helping infants to learn safe water sense. See Recommended Reading for books on this subject.

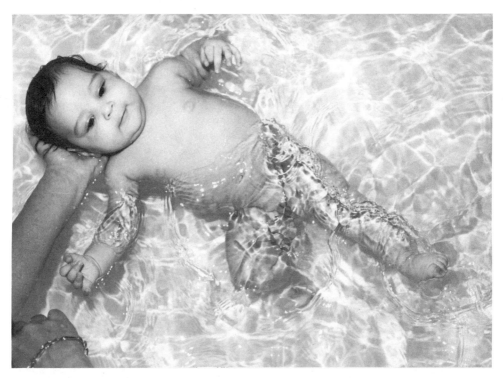

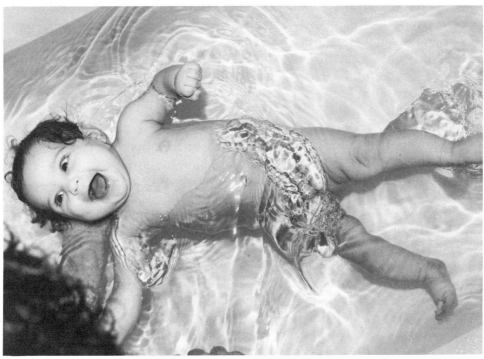

13

Baby Massage

There are many different types of massage, and everyone massages in an individual way. Many mothers intuitively massage their babies from birth. However, modern women seem to have less confidence in their maternal instincts and often appreciate guidance in this special interaction with their infant. This is especially the case if the baby has "colic," poor sleeping patterns, or restlessness.

One way of looking at the types of massage is to categorize the amount of pressure involved. For example, the absolute "lightest" touch would be "unruffling the aura," in which the hands do not touch the body at all but move parallel to the contours a slight distance away from the skin. This type of massage, known as *therapeutic touch*, was pioneered by Dolores Krieger, a professor of nursing at New York University, and is most suitable for a very agitated or restless baby. A regimen using the next level of touch—skin only—has been developed by Ruth Rice, R.N., Ph.D., in Texas, and used successfully with premature babies.

A third level of touch is used by Eva Reich, M.D., and Amelia Auckett, R.N. (the author of *Baby Massage*; see Recommended Reading), who do this massage as a form of therapy as well as pleasurable prevention. This third level moves slightly deeper in that the long muscles of the limbs are gently wobbled, and light finger-circling is done on the body, particularly the belly, shoulders, and back. It is ideal for the first few weeks of life, or at any time to calm a baby.

Finally, a deeper massage, which uses oil and is similar to kneading bread, is done with babies at least one month old. This kind of massage is traditional in India and has been described by Frederic LeBoyer (see Recommended Reading).

I am indebted to Eva Reich for the following massage sequence. Dr. Reich is a pioneer in the field of the physical and emotional environment of babies. This type of massage is designed to soothe and calm both Mother and Baby. It's ideal to do at the end of an exercise session, and can be used for babies of any ages—as long as they lie still! You can continue with this gentle massage for as long as your baby seems to enjoy it, or as Baby gets older you can gradually add more kneading as described in different massage books (see Recommended Reading).

Guidelines for Massaging from Birth to Four Months

Lay your baby on her back on a sheet, blanket, or natural sheepskin in a warm room, or outside if the weather is fine. Undress her completely—massage is much nicer skin-to-skin than through clothes. Leave a diaper under her, though, just in case. In fact, massage is very relaxing and the baby will invariably urinate. Have a blanket nearby to wrap Baby in quickly if she should get tired or hungry.

If your baby seems not to like being undressed, cover the part of her body you are not immediately massaging. Babies soon get used to their "air bath," which is also very nice for their skin, especially in winter.

Newborn babies usually assume a flexed position, so just do as much of the massage as your baby seems to enjoy, increasing at a gradual rate.

Keep your touch *very light*, so that you relax rather than stimulate the baby, especially during the first few weeks. As Eva Reich says, think of touching a butterfly's wings so lightly that you would not rub off any of the texture.

Oil is not necessary with this light, relaxing massage. Using oil would require you to use more pressure with your hands, which is more suited to an older infant than a newborn. The skin of a healthy baby does not need any lotions or potions; in fact, some of them can cause rashes and allergies from the perfumes and other additives. Always avoid what is sold commercially as "baby oil," for this is a petroleum derivative and depletes Baby's body of vitamins A and D. The best oil is cold-pressed and of vegetable origin (such as almond, avocado, or apricot).

You will notice that the stroking movements in the following sequence are always away from the body—drawing off tension. Also, remember, a massage is given as well as received. Make sure you are in a peaceful frame of mind, and in harmony with your baby's mood. Use this sensual interchange to communicate your love and respect to your baby.

An ideal time for either you or your partner to massage your baby is after her bath. Another good time may be before she has a nap. Baby will most likely be quite hungry after her massage and will probably nurse and then enjoy a long sleep.

As your infant grows into a child, she often may not want to lie still for a massage, although some children continue to love being massaged. After the age of about two, your child may want to return the gesture and massage you, especially if she sees you and your partner exchanging massages. The growth of so many massage services in the alternative health community is a response to our continuing need to be touched and our often early deprivation of such communication.

Baby on Her Back

1. Start by making eye contact with your infant and explaining that you are going to have a nice time together for the next few minutes.

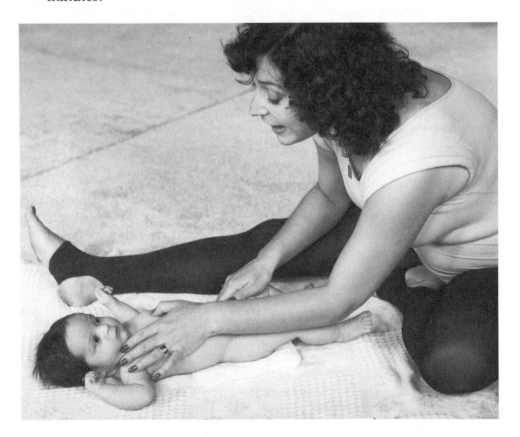

"I just love to give her a massage after her bath. I also try to do a little bit each time I change her."

2. Stroke your baby's head and forehead, and around the ears. Avoid stroking the face on newborns, as they will respond with a rooting reflex (turning their face for the nipple). Older infants enjoy gentle strokes around their eyes and along their jaws. Use your judgment about how much you want to soothe or stimulate your infant.

(continued)

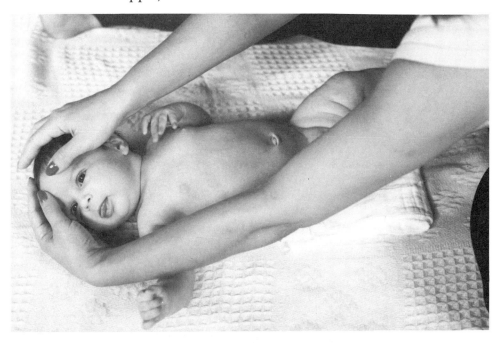

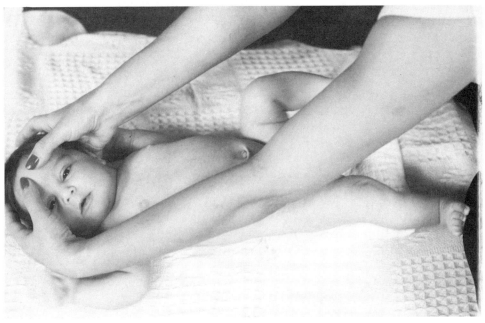

Baby on Her Back (continued)

3. Stroke down Baby's arms—very lightly, as if touching only the skin. Sometimes infants will open their hands and you can stroke the palms and fingers, too. If your baby doesn't, never mind—don't force her hands open, as this just stimulates the grasp reflex.

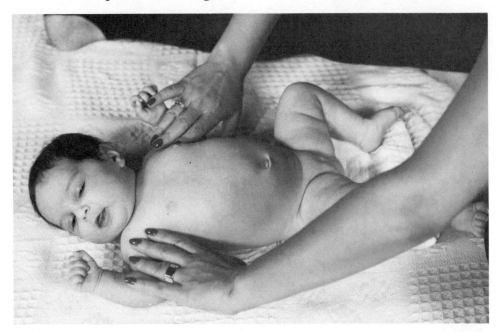

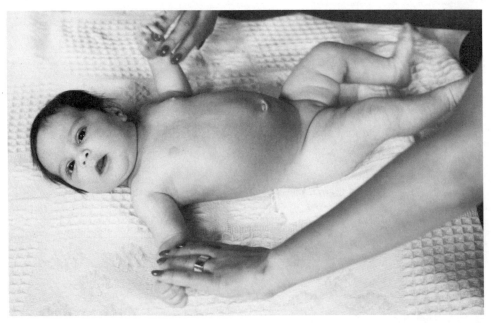

4. Gently wobble the muscles of Baby's upper arms and forearms, just as you would wobble jell-o without breaking it.

(continued)

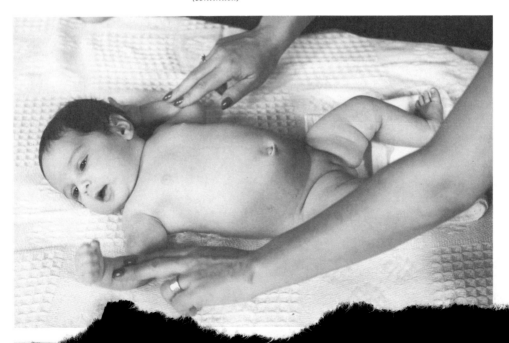

Baby on Her Back (continued)

5. Stroke Baby's chest. Begin with your fingers on Baby's breast-bone and stroke sideways, following the contour of her ribs.

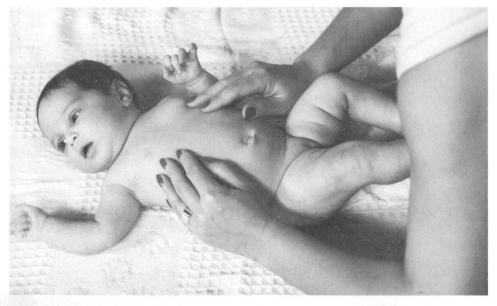

6. Make gentle circles with one fin-
ome of
the

7. Massage Baby's belly with one hand, using your palm. Always move in a clockwise direction, because this is the way the intestines empty.

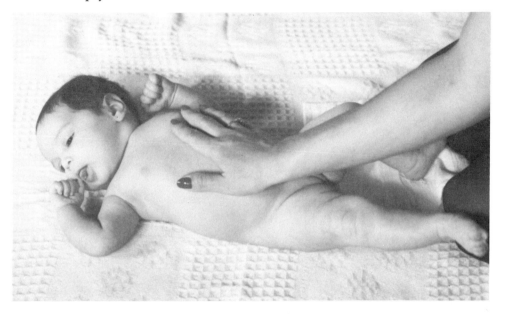

8. Stroke down Baby's legs. Keep your touch as light as a feather.
(continued)

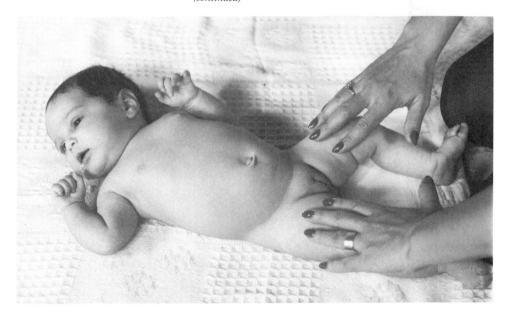

Baby on Her Back (continued)

9. Wobble the muscles of Baby's thighs and calves.

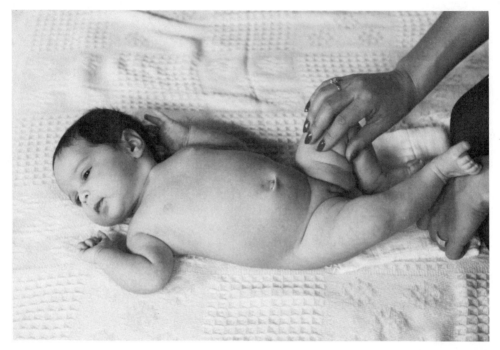

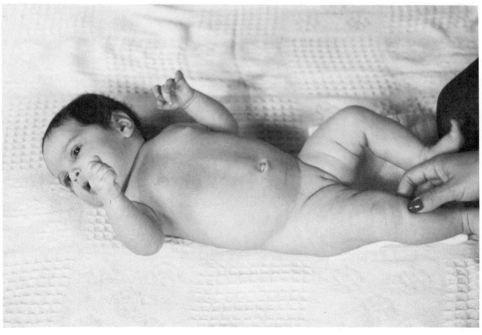

10. Massage Baby's feet, with a firmer touch to avoid tickling. Play with each little toe.

(continued)

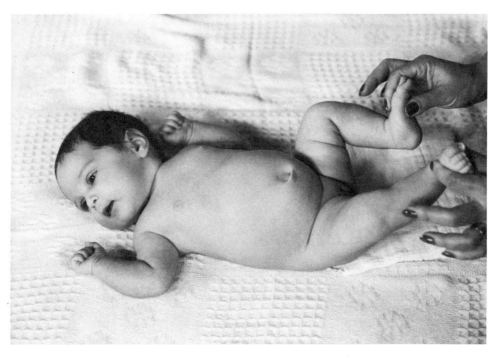

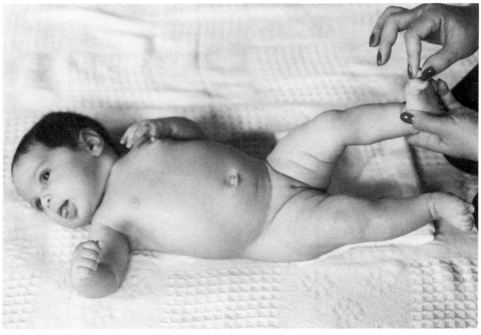

Baby on Her Back (continued)

11. Finish by sweeping your hands lightly over Baby from top to toe, covering as much skin as possible and including her genital area.

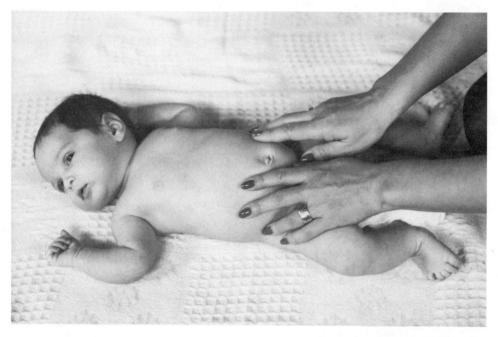

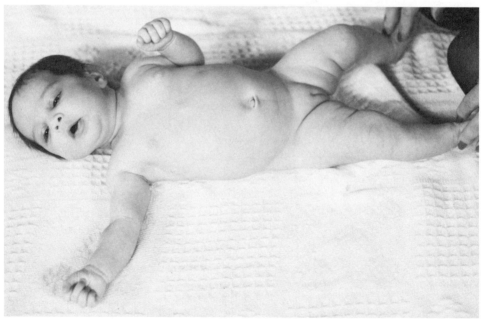

Baby on Her Front

1. Stroke Baby's head, neck (what you can find of it!), and shoulders. Sometimes babies pick up tension in the same area as their mother has it. For example, if you have a tense neck and shoulders, your baby may like some finger-circling in this area.

(continued)

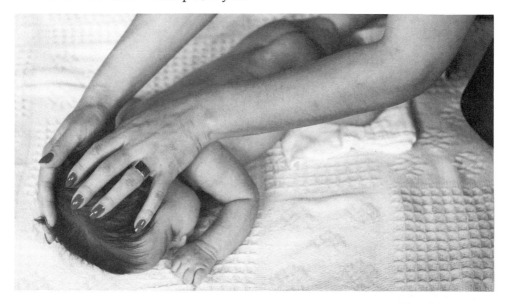

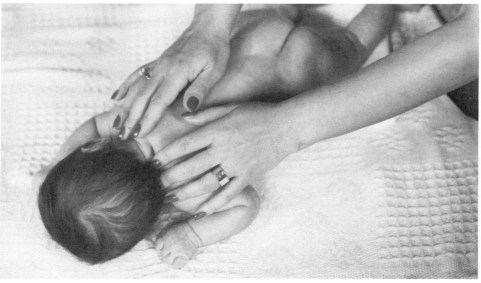

Baby on Her Front (continued)

2. Stroke Baby's back with your palm.

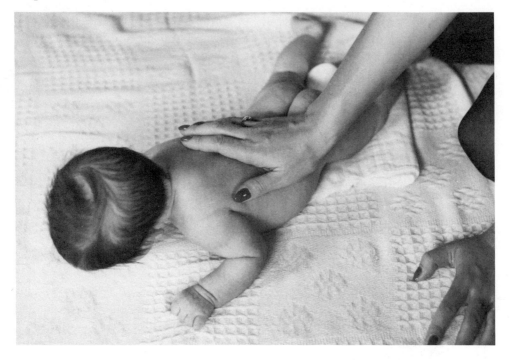

"Remember to keep your touch very light."

3. Stroke with a fingertip down
each side of Baby's spine, or
make a series of little finger circles down each side of the spine.

(continued)

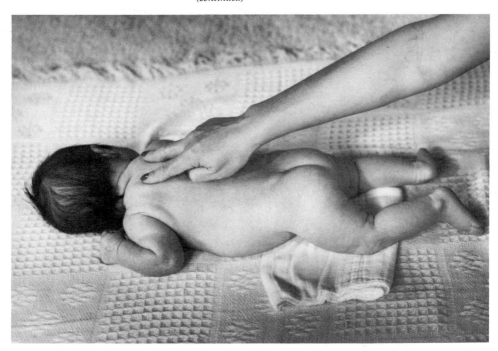

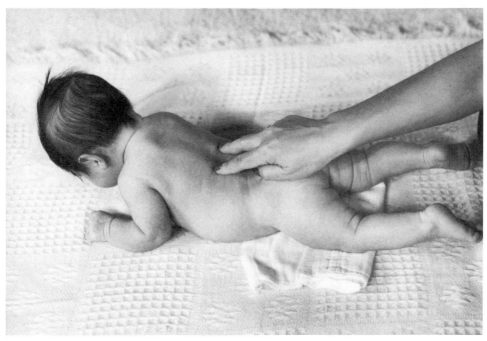

Baby on Her Front (continued)

4. Wobble Baby's buttocks.

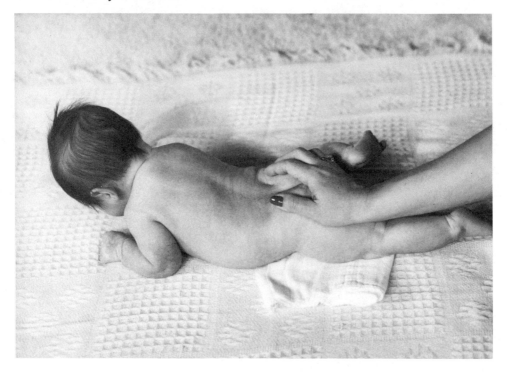

"Try to be sensitive to your baby's mood."

5. Finish by stroking Baby's whole body from crown to toes several times.

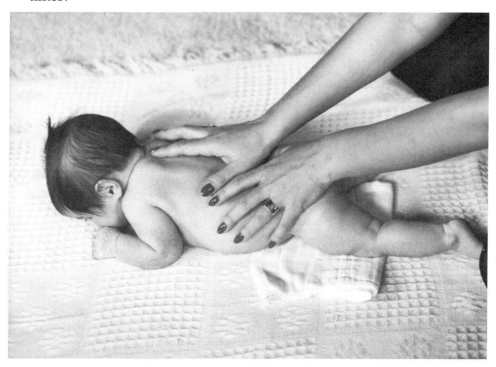

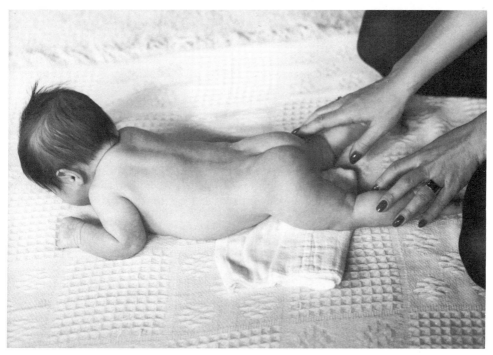

Recommended Reading

Bookstores

The following bookstores specialize in mail-order books on pregnancy, birth, and parenthood. Write for their free, annotated booklists.

Birth and Life Bookstore, P.O. Box 70625, Seattle, WA 98107.

ICEA Bookcenter, P.O. Box 20048, Minneapolis, MN 55420.

John Holt Associates, 729 Boylston Street, Boston, MA 02116. Selected books for children and families, and an annotated booklist.

Journals

Mothering. P.O. Box 2208, Dept. B.L., Albuquerque, NM 97103. A bimonthly magazine dealing with pregnancy, birth, parenthood, and family life. Alternative philosophies, health remedies, and interesting ads for all kinds of products of interest to families.

Postpartum Exercises

Noble, Elizabeth. *Essential Exercises for the Childbearing Year*. 2nd ed., rev. Boston: Houghton Mifflin, 1982. Describes the role of key muscles (the abdominals and pelvic floor) through pregnancy, birth, and postpartum. Emphasizes women's understanding of their bodies. Details preventive and restorative exercises, including after cesarean birth.

Baby Exercises

Barnes, Joan, and Astor, Susan D., with Umberto Tosi. *Gymboree: Giving Your Child Physical, Mental and Social Confidence Through Play*. New York: Dolphin, 1981.

Levy, Janine. *The Baby Exercise Book*. New York: Pantheon, 1973. Detailed exercises for the first fifteen months.

Baby Massage

Auckett, Amelia. *Baby Massage: Parent-Child Bonding Through Touching.* New York: Newmarket, 1982. A sensitive understanding of the energy between parents and baby.

LeBoyer, Frederic. *Loving Hands.* New York: Knopf, 1976. The traditional Indian art of massage for babies aged one month to six months.

Schneider, Vimala. *Infant Massage: A Handbook for Loving Parents.* New York: Bantam, 1982. Describes Indian and Swedish massage techniques, with lullabies to sing during massage.

Breastfeeding

Brewer, Gail Sforza, and Presser, Janice. *Breastfeeding.* New York: Knopf, 1983.

Brewster, Dorothy P. *You Can Breastfeed Your Baby . . . Even in Special Situations.* Emmaus, Penn: Rodale Press, 1979. A complete, well-illustrated reference for situations such as multiple births, prematurity, and surgery.

Bumgarner, Norma Jean. *Mothering Your Nursing Toddler.* Rev. ed. La Leche League International, 9616 Minneapolis Avenue, Franklin Park, IL 60131. An inspiring book for parents of a breastfeeding toddler, with sensitive insights into the needs of children.

La Leche League, International. *The Womanly Art of Breastfeeding.* New York: New American Library, 1984. The classic manual from the international association of nursing mothers.

Pryor, Karen. *Nursing Your Baby.* New York: Pocket Books, 1976. A practical guide for all aspects of breastfeeding.

Raphael, Dana. *Breastfeeding: The Tender Gift.* New York: Schocken, 1977. Describes the support and nurturing necessary for a mother to successfully breastfeed.

Child Care

Brazleton, T. Berry. *On Becoming a Family: The Growth of Attachment.* New York: Delacorte, 1981. A supportive book to help parents stay in love with their babies. Excellent explanations of newborn behavior and interesting family histories.

Brewer, Gail Sforza, and Greene, Janice Presser. *Right from the Start: Meeting the Challenge of Mothering Your Unborn and Newborn Child.* Emmaus, Penn.: Rodale Press, 1981. Sound advice for the immediate postpartum period. Highly recommended.

Jones, Sandy. *To Love a Baby.* Boston: Houghton Mifflin, 1981. A poetic message, with beautiful photographs, exploring parental emotions and attachment to the unborn and newborn baby.

Kenda, Margaret E., and Williams, Phyllis S. *The Natural Baby Food Cookbook.* New York: Avon, 1972. Good information and recipes for providing your growing infant with healthful food.

Klaus, Marshall H., and Kennell, John H. *Parent-Infant Bonding*. Rev. ed. St. Louis: Mosby, 1982. A revision and expansion of the original pioneering studies on human attachment to the newborn.

Leach, Penelope. *Your Baby and Child*. New York: Random House, 1980. A comprehensive guide to all aspects of child care in the first five years.

Samuels, Mike, and Samuels, Nancy. *The Well Baby Book*. New York: Summit, 1979. A holistic reference book for the early years.

Wallerstein, Edward. *Circumcision: An American Health Fallacy*. New York: Springer, 1980. A thoroughly researched investigation into the medically unnecessary practice of circumcision.

White, Burton. *The First Three Years of Life*. New York: Avon, 1978. A developmental guide by a well-known child health specialist.

Dental Care

Moss, Stephen. *Your Child's Teeth*. Boston: Houghton Mifflin, 1980. Stresses preventive dental hygiene beginning with Baby's first tooth.

Swimming

Sidenbladh, Erik. *Water Babies*. New York: St. Martin's Press, 1982. A fascinating description of Russian experiments with humans and animals in water.

Timmermans, Claire. *How to Teach Your Baby to Swim,* New York: Stein and Day, 1975. A step-by-step, illustrated guide for pool activities.

Family Relationships

Farson, Richard. *Birthrights*. New York: Macmillan, 1974. Exciting new ideas.

Friday, Nancy. *My Mother, My Self*. New York: Dell, 1978. A penetrating and absorbing book dealing with all levels of mother-daughter relationships.

Fromm, Erich. *The Art of Loving: An Enquiry into the Nature of Love*. New York: Harper and Row, 1965. A cultural, philosophical, and psychological discussion of the value and expression of love.

Janov, Arthur. *The Feeling Child*. New York: Simon and Schuster, 1975. The importance of freedom and acceptance in the development of a child's "real" self. How to avoid inducing fear, tension, conflict, and neurosis in children.

La Leche League, International. *The Heart Has Its Reasons*. New York: New American Library, 1985. For mothers who choose to stay home with their children.

Liedloff, Jean. *The Continuum Concept*. New York: Warner, 1972. How children are happier, more relaxed, and more independent in cultures where they experience much body contact and share adult lives—always present, but never the center of attention.

Montagu, Ashley. *Touching: The Human Significance of the Skin.* Rev. ed. New York: Perennial, 1978. An anthropological view of physical intimacy within families, and child-raising practices. Discusses swaddling, rocking, breastfeeding.

Prescott, James W. "Body Pleasure and the Origins of Violence," *Bulletin of the Atomic Scientists.* November 1975. A neuropsychologist contends that the greatest threat to world peace comes from those nations that have the most depriving environments for their children and that are most repressive of sexual expression, particularly female sexuality.

Thevenin, Tine. *The Family Bed—An Age Old Concept in Childrearing.* Available from the bookstores listed above or from the author at P.O. Box 16004, Minneapolis, MN 55416. A convincing argument for the family's sleeping together.

Learning Versus Education

Read these books while your child is still an infant—they will help you to explore your values and philosophy about discipline.

Holt, John. *How Children Learn.* New York: Dell, 1967. A former schoolteacher shows how conventional education is ineffective and degrading. Describes how children figure out the world for themselves through play and motivation.

Neill, A. S. *Summerhill: A Radical Approach to Child Rearing.* New York: Pocket Books, 1977. Observations of a pioneering British educator and original thinker on the needs of children for freedom, responsibility, and creativity.

Pierce, Joseph Chilton. *Magical Child.* New York: Dutton, 1977. On self-worth.

Stallibrass, Alison. *The Self-Respecting Child.* New York: Warner, 1979. A fascinating account of the structure and importance of children's spontaneous play for all aspects of development.

Resources

American Foundation for Maternal and Child Health, Inc., 30 Beekman Place, New York, NY 10022. Information and resources.

American Holistic Medical Association, 6932 Little River Turnpike, Annandale, VA 22003. Referrals to alternative physicians.

Association for Parents of Children with Learning Disabilities (ACLD), 1456 Library Road, Pittsburgh, PA 15236. Provides information on helping children with normal intelligence overcome or cope with learning, perceptual, and/or behavioral handicaps.

Center for the Study of Multiple Birth, Suite 463-5, 333 East Superior Street, Chicago, IL 60611. Provides information on the risks and special problems encountered in twin and other multiple pregnancies. Mail-order bookstore.

Closer Look, Box 1492, Washington D.C. 20013. Information on services and financial assistance for parents of children with all types of handicaps.

International Childbirth Education Association (ICEA), P.O. Box 20048, Minneapolis, MN 55420. An umbrella organization providing information on all aspects of pregnancy, birth, and parenthood, with a specialized mail-order bookcenter.

La Leche League International, 9616 Minneapolis Avenue, Franklin Park, IL 60131. A volunteer organization of mothers with local chapters throughout the U.S. offering support and counseling for breasfeeding. Information pamphlets and nursing aids.

Maternal and Child Health Center, 2464 Massachusetts Avenue, Cambridge, MA 02140. A resource center for pregnancy, birth, and postpartum. Classes in prenatal and postpartum exercise, preparation for natural childbirth and parenthood, groups for mothers with infants and crawlers. Library, referrals, labor support, and individual counseling and therapy.

National Organization of Mothers of Twins Clubs, Inc., 5402 Amberwood Lane, Rockville, MD 20853. Information on state and local chapters. Publishes a quarterly newsletter and several information booklets.

The Children's Foundation, 1521 16th Street N.W., Washington D.C. 20036. Information on food programs such as WIC (Women, Infants, and Children) supplements.

Vaginal Birth After Caesarean (VBAC), 10 Great Plain Terrace, Needham, MA 02192. For information, send a stamped, self-addressed envelope and $1 c/o Nancy Cohen.

Index